# THE PLEASURES
# OF **TESTICLES:**

*A Celebration and Exploration of*
## ALL THINGS BALLS

# JAMES L. RIEDY

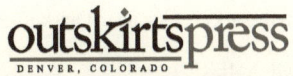

outskirtspress
DENVER, COLORADO

Outskirts Press, Inc.
http://www.outskirtspress.com

ISBN: 978-1-4327-8889-6

Outskirts Press and the "OP" logo are trademarks belonging to Outskirts Press, Inc.

# Table of Contents

# Preface

At long last! A general-interest book about balls, meaning testicles:

*Hairy, dangling orbs, loose, tight, pendulous, shaved or plain, with eggs, containing the future. Fearsome in their delicacy, flotsam & jetsam. Pull them, prod them, flaunt, implore, tickle. Adore the balls.*

There are approximately six billion of them on our planet, each set pumping out daily over 96 million sperm — some of the most extraordinary cells of the body, a triumph of efficient packaging, sleek design, and super specialization.

This exploration comes at a moment in American history when the male is feeling threatened as never before. His pride, his self-esteem, his sense of superiority are being diminished by a multiplicity of forces beyond his control. He is increasingly genetically expendable. Professor Greg Stock declares that the concept of having sex in order to create kiddies will be dead within twenty years. Genes researcher Jennifer A. Marshall Graves in Australia argues for eventual extinction of the Y chromosome. "Advances in cryogenics and turkey basting have rendered human males largely superfluous," writes Donald G. McNeil, Jr. As though this weren't enough, Peter McAllister, another

Australian, provides a bracing portrait of masculinity in decline in his new book *Manthropology: The Science of Why the Modern Male Is Not the Man He Used to Be*. In the fall of 2012 Riverhead Books published Hanna Rosin's provocative *The End of Men: And the Rise of Women*--"Men are losing their grip, patriarchy is crumbling." Several new sitcoms make fun of men, so much so that the word *man* itself is treated as a joke. Take two that premiered in 2011: *Man Up!* and ABC's other emasculation comedy, *Last Man Standing*. Earlier P. D. James published his novel, *The Children of Men,* set in a future where the world's male population becomes infertile and state-run "national porn shops" stimulate the flagging male libido.

Further support for a book such as this one is the increased attention being directed to the human body and to certain of its parts. "Once more," acknowledges *The New York Times*, "that which was private has become public. Gradually, references to men's genitals — their images and functions — have been permeating popular culture." An issue of the remarkably successful *Men's Health* magazine published a guide to "understanding, maintaining and trouble shooting that holiest of appliances, your privates."

Morrow, Taschen, and St. Martin's have published general-appeal books on the penis. Steven Vaschon released *Rear View*, his debut collection of black-and-white photographs featuring male backsides.

In 2000 Rebecca Chalker explored women's genital anatomy and ways for women to increase their sexual response in her book *The Clitoral Truth: The Secret World at Your Fingertips*. Six years later the travelling Vulva Museum Exhibit/Speaker Event was launched. The museum included positive vulva imagery in art, jewelry, sculpture, graphic art and more. The following year Penguin released *Body Drama*, a sassy photographic body manual that included an array of two dozen vulvas of diverse colors and grooming persuasions. In 2008 Richard Beck Peacock created *Petals: A Journey Into Self-Discovery*, a 49-minute documentary of Nick Karras's stunning, tastefully shot photographic studies of 48 vulvas.

Bigger things were to follow: *Vulvagraphics: An Intervention in Honor of Female Genital Diversity*, a preeminent art show displaying "the beauty and diversity of vulvas," opened in New York, fall of 2009. That same year Naomi Wolf signed on with Ecco Press for a project titled *Vagina: A Cultural History*. Two years later Hylton Coxwell put together a vast array of photos for his coffee table book *Vulva 101*, Show Off Books released *I'll Show You Mine*, personal stories and photos — unaltered, life-sized, and life color, of 60 women's genitals, and artist Jamie McCartney was creating his 29-foot-long "Great Wall of Vagina" — 400 plaster casts of vulvas (all of them unique).

With the external genitals of females getting so much attention the thought was beginning to permeate: what about the slighted testicles — dismissed, undervalued, unexplored, and misunderstood?

By now almost everyone's heard about Eve Ensler's 1998 compilation *The Vagina Monologues*. "When one of the [Vagina] monologues expressed the hope of similarly liberating their testicular brethren," wrote F. Lomax, "I realized why the good Lord had put me on this world equipped with a set of testicles. I got right to work." The end result: a one-man comedy entitled *The Testicular Monologues*.

In Susan Patron's *The Higher Power of Lucky*, which won a prestigious children's literature award, the young readers read: "Scrotum sounded to Lucky like something green that comes up when you have the flu and cough too much. It sounded medical and secret, but also important." A resulting controversy led to an explosion in scrotal-related newspaper stories.

Comedy Central's website launched the animated series *Baxter & McGuire*, about two of the closest of pals, who just happen to be testicles. "I had a ball watching these cohorts do what they have to do to enjoy everyday living in a sticky situation," writes one critic.

In the first episode of the infamous *Ren & Stimpy*, an adult-audience cartoon about a demented Chihuahua and a brain-dead cat duo, whose exploits first aired in 2003, testicles are prominently featured, along with a hairy man's ass, and "Z-cup breasts bounce ad nauseam."

Reflecting on the HBO drama *Tell Me You Love Me*, Sara Vilkomerson observes: "A seismic shift is occurring across the entertainment landscape: men are dropping trou, and penises and testicles are seemingly everywhere, flapping in the breeze." She goes on to ask, "Is the scrotum the new cleavage?" Vilkomerson mentions that audiences literally howled while watching the scandalous *Borat* scene when Ken Davitian's scrotum practically suffocated Sacha Baron Cohen during their naked wrestling match.

The raunchy, lowbrow PG-13 comedy *Balls of Fury,* which opened in theaters late in 2007, provides a steady stream of innuendos about testicles of various shapes and sizes.

Then there's John Barnard's surreal animation, *Testicle Chin Man*, featuring a super hero with balls for a face, and a Peter Farrelly-directed comedy sketch, *The Catch*, starring Hugh Jackman as a man whose testicles are located under his chin.

South African rocker Dave Matthews secured himself a movie production deal "by grabbing his testicles on American TV." More recently the animated TV sitcom *South Park* got away with showing giant testicles.

Boston area artist Jesa Damora (aka Belle Wether) turns out poster-sized black-and-white pencil portraitures of testicles (scrota, actually), capturing every nook, cranny, and ridge in stunning photorealistic detail. The cost: $5,000 plus tax, shipping, and insurance.

The dinner table centerpieces at an elaborate show in the Big Apple benefiting Broadway Cares/Equity Fights AIDS were loaves of bread "shaped like oversize genitals," and along with the meat entrée were "potatoes positioned like low dropping testicles."

Beyond mere suggestion, there's testicle pizza and testicle goulash, as detailed in Serbian chef Ljubomir Erovic's *The Testicle Cookbook: Cooking With Balls*.

Former Hewlett-Packard Co. CEO Carly Fiorina, during a meeting at her earlier tech company, Lucent Technologies, showed up with two pairs of her husband's socks stuffed in her trousers, and told the audience, "Our balls are as big as anyone's in this room."

Driving around the USA, you'll see "truck nuts" — a plastic or metal novelty item resembling testicles, found dangling from the bumpers of pickup trucks, Jeeps, and ATVs. BullsBalls.com, for one, has about 500 distributors and grosses close to $1 million a year for its "made to swing" accessories, while Your Nutz, a San Diego business, sells over 200 kinds of fake testicles. Another company introduces Ballsies, "the first line of jewelry that captures the essence of everyone's favorite baggy buddies." The sterling silver testicle necklaces for women, priced at $54.95, come packaged "in our sweet Ballsies tin and pink ultra-suede pouch."

Winning the Grabby Award for the Best Comedy of 2010 was *Whorrey Potter and the Sorcerer's Balls*, a gay parody of *Harry Potter and the Sorcerer's Stone*.

Despite their vulnerability and unprepossessing appearance (Sylvia Plath in *The Bell Jar* compares them to "turkey gizzards," and Camille Paglia in her tome *Sexual Personai* calls them ludicrous because of their "rubbery indecisiveness"), balls have occupied a critical place in our culture. Or consider the words of the eighteenth-century French friar and philosophy professor Joseph Galien: *Les testicules sont précieux que le Coeur lui-même; le Coeur n'est utile que pour vivre, tandis que les testicules le sont pour bien vivre.* ["Testicles are more precious than the heart itself; the heart is only useful for living, but the testicles are for living well."]

According to AdultGroupRepertory.com, "the largest repository of Yahoo! adult groups on the Web," in 2010 over 500 of the more than 175,000 adult content Yahoo! groups (an Internet communication tool) were dedicated to them: Knackerbag has over 3100 members who admit that "a big pair of bull balls, hangin' heavy and low in a loose, fleshy ball sac is a fine sight to behold in a man." Low Hangers, with over 8800 members, is devoted to "our interest in, fascination of, appreciation for, and love of guys' balls — the very best, most beautiful, delicious and wonderful part of the male body."

Great Ballz, another website, gives subscribers who pay $9.95 a month access to more than 1200 pictures of "the biggest, plumpest, juiciest, bounciest balls anywhere."

Testicles, a similar site, "was created due to the lack of existing materials that focus solely on one of the most erotic and overlooked parts of the male anatomy ... testicles."

Finally, not overlooking them is the daedalian cosmetic industry: Bálla ball powder for men, "the ultimate men's anti-wetness solution," comes unscented, scented with oak and musk, or as a minty and tingly powder. There's also Fresh Balls, a talc-free solution "to keep your boys fresh all day every day."

In 2009 Governor Arnold Schwarzenegger of California, who had warned lawmakers they needed to act boldly and make some tough budget choices, sent Senate president pro-tem Darrell Steinberg a football-sized sculpture of testicles.

That same year it was reported that Stanford researchers had isolated powerful stem cells from human testes and said the cells could ultimately yield a wide variety of human tissues, including cells of the nervous system, the liver, heart, skin, and blood vessels.

"Everywhere you go nowadays, people are talking about testicles," quips Comedy Network's Jon Dore.

Now there is a book about one tantalizing aspect of them: the boundless possibilities for providing pleasure.

I'm enormously grateful to my friends, colleagues, companions, and my beloved ballsy mother, all of whom assisted in a variety of ways in helping to bring this book finally to fruition. Specifically: Edmund J. Dehnert and Don Smith, members of the City Colleges of Chicago Humanities Department; Frank Williams, who edited my earlier book; Victor Matus, who never ceased urging me onward; and friend John Charles, whose erudition and insightful suggestions were enormously beneficial. Additional gratitude is extended to some national organizations that invited me to give presentations at their annual conventions: The American Urological Association, The American Culture Association, and The Society for the Scientific Study of Sexuality.

# CHAPTER 1

# Aesthetic Pleasures

Beyond satisfying a man sexually, do women have any prurient interest in the testes? In *Dick Talk*, an anonymously produced video by some women in the Houston area (available through the Houston Center for Photography where it was once shown), one participant forthrightly expresses a preference for "a good set of balls." And *Playgirl* magazine's Vivian Holland, remarking spiritedly about film star Matthew Modine's endowments as noticed in the shower scene of Robert Altman's movie *Streamers*, talks about the actor's "two bounteous balls."

Writing for Salon.com, Harriet Archer, in her article, "Baseball Is the Sexiest Sport," discloses: "When women speak of baseball players, we tend to talk of tight pants, of bats and balls, of butts and backs and biceps.... We giggle when the guys rearrange their testicles."

Anne MacNaughton, whose celebratory poem, "Teste Moanial," is included in *The Best American Poetry, 1989*, rhapsodizes: "Actually, it's the balls I look for, always." She continues:

Men in the street, offices, cars, restaurants,
it's the nuts I imagine —
firm, soft, in hairy sacks
the way they are

down there rigged between the thighs,
the funny way they are.
One in front, a little in front of the other,
slightly higher. The way they slip
between your fingers, the way they
slip around in their soft sack.
The way they swing when he walks,
hang down when he bends
over. You see them sometimes bright pink
out of a pair of shorts
when he sits wide and unaware,
the hair sparse and wiry
like that on a Poland china pig.
You can see the skin right through — speckled,
with wrinkles like a prune, but loose,
slipping over those kernels
rocking the smooth, small huevos.
So delicate, the cock becomes a diversion,
a masthead overlarge, its flag distracting
from beautiful pebbles beneath.

The variety of sexual practices for gratification's sake involving the testicles is seemingly without limits. "I don't have a huge repertoire," confides Josey Vogels in her online "My Messy Bedroom" column. "I've obviously been missing out. I found all kinds of things online that one can do with balls that I'd never even imagined."

## To Shave or Not

In *Playgirl* magazine a New York man (name withheld) reported that his girlfriend "lovingly removed the hair at the base of my cock and all from the scrotum." He continued: "We go through the ceremony every week or so, keeping my balls as satiny smooth as they were when they dropped in the sack at age thirteen. My girl says it's a real turn-on for her to shave them, and I confess that I get hot as hell while she does it. The aftermath is explosive."

Responding to that letter, a woman from the other end of the nation wrote that she finds a hairy scrotum "incredibly sexy."

Freelancer Bryce Van Hoosen concedes that some women will tell you that shaved balls are unappealing, resembling a saggy turkey sack. Since there are those who are so repulsed by testicle hair, Van Hoosen suggests a way to please every taste: shave one ball and let the other one grow.

For those preferring the clean-shaven look, there are a number of "personal" shavers on the market. Bodworx International promotes its "scientifically designed lite-weight testicle shaver [that] changes the way you remove unwanted hair." The Body Bare pubic shaver "will not ever nick or scrape your skin," and comes with a lifetime guarantee. After the shaving, one product recommended is Balla Powder for men: "asbestos free and feels like you have an air conditioner in your underwear."

Just how common are clean-shaven balls? By 2011, Yahoo! was providing over 62,000 entries dealing with scrotum grooming. Bing had over 77,000. Among them: "Shaving isn't a 'gay thing.' It's a male thing. One straight man I know shaves himself and his wife says that aside from the kink value, it makes sex a bit more interesting." Another writes: "After the first shave I was hooked. The smooth feel of my balls was worth all the effort; they were awesome. I couldn't believe I hadn't uncovered those beauties before. The sensitivity went through the roof, and the wife said sucking them was a treat. All I needed to hear shaving equals better blow jobs, sold." And: "All chicks dig ... shaved nuts. When your balls are shaved women are more apt to muzzling [sic] your jewels with their lovely mouths." "I've never met a woman who didn't appreciate the clean look of shaved junk."

Simlar testimonials appear on the website unabashedly named I Shave My Balls -- "true personal stories from a group of people who all say, 'I Shave My Balls.' Sign up takes just seconds, so join today!"

One member writes: "I keep my balls smooth so that when they dangle I can see all of the wrinkles and the firm balls within."

"Squirm all you like. There's an immense subculture of eroticists who claim a bald bag makes for better sex," admits James Whittall, president of MenEssentials.

In her book *Doing It — Real People Having Really Good Sex* Isadora Alman quotes a woman: "There is nothing like the feel of those smooth, freshly shaved balls. I could stay there forever, just rubbing my nose, mouth, and cheek against them. Feeling them in my hands is a very lovely experience. I love the feel of those smooth balls!"

Sexologist Alman in her syndicated advice column "Ask Isadora" responded to the following query about scrotum shaving:

I've noticed that a lot of men in gay porn have their scrotums (scrota?) shaved. I like the look and would like to try it myself. However, the idea of getting a razor near my balls is very frightening. Do you know how to get rid of the hair with as little pain and danger to possible? I know I could ask some other man about this, but I'm new to the life and would be very embarrassed. Plus I think it's a little kinky. I can only deal with one new bit of self-disclosure in public at a time.

Isadora's advice:

Not being one to be daunted by embarrassment or kink, I asked someone well-versed in the process. My friend James says that 'due to testicular typography, shaving the scrotum is really best done as a three handed process.' He suggests (and others concur) sitting in a bathtub with a well-lathered subject at hand, loosened and relaxed. One person uses two hands to stretch the skin flat and the other uses a disposable safety razor or two or three. This is not a straight blade, so there is no risk of castration.

The worst that can happen is a surface skin nick handleable [sic] with styptic pencil or Betadine. If the assistance of a very good friend is too much to ask for, depilatories aimed at women's bikini areas are designed for very sensitive skin.

JustUsBoys, "The World's Largest Gay Porn Portal," online since mid-2002 and claiming over 138,000 members in 2012, reported these results of its Bald Balls poll: "I shave my balls," 65%; "Are you crazy! The family jewels are best untouched," 20%; "I prefer my man to have shaved, clean balls," 32%; "The more hair the better. Also serves as flossing," 7%.

Online sassy expert Josey Vogels, Canada's premier sex and relationship columnist, reports that the owner of an electrology clinic in Vancouver "zaps the genitals of two to three men a day." The procedure is neither cheap nor fast. It costs about $60 an hour, and to permanently remove the hair at the base of the penis and the scrotum will take several sessions over a couple years for a total cost of between $2000 and $3000.

References to shaved balls abound in first-person narratives on Google's gay sex stories group site: "Meanwhile I was fondling his chest and running my hands down round his newly **shaved balls**." "Tom, remember I asked earlier if you would show me how to shave my balls? I find the idea of having **shaved balls** very erotic." "My boyish cock drips and trembles as I stroke my **shaved balls** with the other hand." "As his cock softened I was able to take his entire manhood into my mouth until my nose pressed into his **shaved balls**."

Every issue of *Smooth Buddies Bulletin*, a now-defunct quarterly journal self-described as "the body shaver's resource, contact, and information," carried over 40 columns of personal ads, many mentioning shaved testicles. "Looking to meet cute GWM [gay white male] about my age and build (not too heavy) with nice shaved balls — and more." "There's nothing as erotic for me as a pair of shaved balls except a pair needing to be shaved."

One member of the Shaved Buddies fraternity gave these details: "Recently I started tweezering [sic] my balls and now the hairs grow back very, very lightly — almost gone. I like to let my hair grow back, then take my trusty Wahl clipper and take it all off near the skin and keep the resulting clipping in a plastic Ziploc bag."

In a "Making It Smooth" article — "a compilation of letters from Smooth Buddies members about their own personal shaving techniques" — one writer disclosed that for about a year he was the "official shaver" at Pork, New York City's "hot leather bar"; he "shaved everything and every type of guy over the course of that year."

The protagonist in "The Styling Salon," a short story in an issue of *Smooth Buddies Bulletin* by a Tampa, FL member who himself did body grooming — "relaxing, sensual, erotic, and fun" — describes this moment: "The razor moved down the back of my balls, dangerously, agonizingly, gently making them smoother and smoother. 'Okay,' he said, 'turn back over.' He then lathered my balls up and shaved the remaining hair from my balls."

Among products especially recommended for scrotum shaving is SensaShave Rash Free 6 Ounce Body Shave Cream For Men: "No bumps. No irritations. No rashes. Just soft, silky smooth skin all around your genital area for your partner." Says *Sex in Review*, a free online magazine of consumer information on sex-related products and services launched in 2000, "It is a basic truth that shaved balls get played with and licked more. Unless your partner has a hairy testicles fetish, chances are that keeping them shaved smooth is going to get them a lot more attention. Of course, you can use regular shaving cream. However, I think the blade glides a little easier across those delicate areas when you use SensaShave."

The current trend, according to hearsay, appeared first as a common beauty treatment for gay men. Someone has written: "I have always heard that what the gay male community wears and does in NY, LA and London filters slowly enough down through society." Says one well-known Manhattan businessman: "I have no f*cking idea why you gay guys are so into that godawful Danish modern furniture. But I've totally gotta give it up to you on the ball-waxing. Wow! What a brilliant invention." Of course, ancient Roman men also removed their body hair to signify their distinction from barbarians and to inscribe culture, as opposed to nature, on their bodies.

Regarding the new wave of male clients, one New York aesthetician admitted to *Newsweek* in 2006, "It's not their backs I'm waxing. It's their balls."

A year later *The New York Observer*'s Simon Doonan wrote:

> This trend for scrotal depilatory procedures — they call it 'manscaping' — has now gone way beyond the confines of Chelsea. Top Manhattan dermatologist Brad Katchen has seen a surge of interest from this unexpected quarter. 'Those Wall Street guys who used to just get their backs lasered are now requesting the genital area. They have developed an interest in aesthetics.'

One Montreal waxophile admitted that his girlfriend is an enthusiastic supporter of the practice. "I'm the first guy she's gone out with who does this. At first she asked why I do it. Now she asks when I'm going to get it done again."

Another guy says he gets plenty of comments about his hairless pair. "The girls really like it. They just think it's great. And they're more willing to pay a lot of special attention to that area. If you know what I mean."

## Piercing

An additional trendy practice among heterosexuals, although more common in the gay community, is scrotal piercing. Writes one

BME [Body Modification Ezine] reader:

> It all started when my wife asked for a navel piercing for her birthday. About 6 months later I decided I wanted a piercing, too. Because of my job I really couldn't get something that was visible, so something under my clothes was necessary. I'd been looking at BME for a few months and decided that a scrotal piercing was for me. The day finally came. We picked out a 12-gauge ring; I figured I could go bigger, but going smaller would be more difficult. I walked into the room, which looks very much like a doctor's or dentist's office. We sat down with the piercer, the same one who did my wife's navel and nipples, so I was pretty comfortable with him. He explained exactly what he was going to do and what I could expect; and showed me all the instruments.

The writer concludes: "I love my scrotal ring, so does my wife. She's constantly playing with it. Actually we both constantly play with it. We were at a party with some of her friends recently and they wanted to see my piercing. Of course, I showed it to them. My wife told them all how much she loves pulling it."

Body piercing has always been "more heavy in the S/M gay part of society," said a senior piercer at Gauntlet Enterprises, the company that pioneered body piercing in North America. Founded in November 1975 by internationally known piercing authority Jim Ward, its customers originally came from a group of gay Los Angeles men known as the P&T Group [for Pierced and Tattooed]. Ward later opened stores in San Francisco and New York. He once estimated he had pierced "several hundred scrotums." Preferring to think of piercing as "a sensual conscious-raising ritual," Ward once told this author about one man whose scrotum was bedecked with 100 rings that were inserted over several years.

BME, the online site famous for its coverage of extreme body modification, printed an account from one gay man entitled "My Road to 12 Scrotal Piercings." "With all these piercings my sack now resides forward and higher up to the penis. It is such a rush. Makes me look hung more than I am. Sex has become much more pleasurable. The slapping of the rings and the pulling back on the skin makes the orgasms last longer and much more intense." He confides: "Ninety percent of my straight friends have genital piercing; less than twenty percent of my gay friends."

Another gay man wrote to BME: "For me piercings are definitely attractive, but more than anything else a way to express myself and an important part of my sexual life."

Scrotum piercings may be placed in a variety of configurations and gauges. The most common are done horizontally at a minimum of 12 gauge. Although the vertical placement is uncommon, they have been done successfully with straight and curved barbells.

Celebrated piercer Elayne Angel, president of the Association of Professional Piercers, founder of Rings of Desire, Inc. in the French Quarter of New Orleans and earlier vice-president of Gauntlet's Southern California operation, is credited with inventing, naming, and popularizing a number of specific piercing placements including the "lorum" — a piercing placed horizontally on the underside of the penis at its base where penis meets scrotum. "I'm sure I've done in the hundreds of scrotum piercings over the years," she said. Her book *The Piercing Bible — The Definitive Guide to Safe Body Piercing* offers details on scrotum piercing, placement, and choice of jewelry.

Another procedure — transscrotal piercing — travels through the scrotum from front to back. A complex piercing and potentially dangerous, it is humorously referred to as a *scrunnel* [short for scrotal tunnel].

Tasha Berg, partner with her husband of the nationally patronized piercing shop Pins and Needles (established in 1992 in Tampa, FL), who learned the technique from Ward, recalled her very first piercing job: the appendage of a scrotal sac. Since then both she and her husband had pierced dozens.

In his short story, "My Testicles Are De Happy Color of De Coco Bean," author Michael Smith, winner of the 1994 Tulsa Library Short Fiction Award, writes:

> It's amazing what can sneak past one's consciousness in the midst of a vacation, under the spell of the tropic sun — an elderly man who must have been in his seventies shuffling around the beach with about nine tinky padlocks hanging from his scrotum. He sported no blue Mohawk, nor was his hair spiked. He appeared a normal old guy who could have been tottering toward the corner grocery for a newspaper instead of down the white sand toward the grass hut/bar. Except, of course, he was naked, as nearly every one at the resort was.

In another area of the world the *hafada*, part of the puberty rites of several Arab tribes in the Persian Gulf region, involves inserting a gold or silver ring through the side of the scrotum between the testicle and the base of the penis. This is intended to prevent the testicles from ever rising back into the body, thus ensuring that the youth will forever be a man.

Besides the piercings already mentioned, there are temporary or play piercings of the testes described in s/m circles as "VERY heavy head trips." The "perfect" instrument is a sterile hypodermic needle. Instructions were detailed in an issue of *Dungeon Master*:

> The testicles must be completely immobilized in the scrotum, either by spreading on a butterfly board or by other forms of bondage. The scrotal skin must be cleaned and only a sterile hypodermic needle used. The needle should be plunged slowly and steadily directly into the testicle. It should not go far enough to penetrate the opposite side of the testicle. It is essential that the needle go straight in; it can stay there as

long as you wish, and then come straight out. The tiny size of the needle will do only insignificant damage to the glandular tissue of the testicle if it is not moved about when in place. However, if it is wiggled or manipulated it will act like a stirring rod and cause a great deal of testicular damage.

Beyond being an advanced s/m specialty play piercing has been ardently described as one of the most fascinating forms of body modification. But what does it feel like when having it done? By piercing and stretching the skin endorphins [natural pain killers in the brain] are released that can make the experience remarkably pleasurable and blur the ever tenuous lines between pleasure and pain. The actual hurt has been compared to that of a minor injection. "Looking down and seeing yourself pierced," someone has written, "is just as powerful as the sensation. The visual power of it is amazing."

## Low Hanging

Someone sends this message to lowhangers@yahoogroups.com: "I am 29 y.o. looking for buddies who know how to stretch their nut sack so that it hangs. I get really excited by this, and would like to get mine to hang low."

Popularly termed "hanging heavy" when the testicles are hanging low, the condition gives the cherished impression of an increased sense of masculinity.

The owner of The Male Sack blog appeals to viewers: "Please showcase a nice, low hanging pair of nuts. This is a MUST, since this is what the blog is about. I will not post pics of tight sacks or balls tied up in any way. They must hang freely. The more pics you send the better!"

Why the gonads — so defenseless and vulnerable -- dangle to begin with has inspired several possible theories. One of the more fanciful is that perhaps they evolved in the same spirit as peacock feathers.

In explaining "Why do human testicles hang like that?" a research psychologist writing for *Scientific American* remarks: "Perhaps scrotal testicles evolved as a sort of ornamental display communicating the genetic quality of the male."

The subject has staggering interest. As of early 2012, the search engine Bing provided over two million entries dealing with testicle stretching.

The maximum length of stretch possible is unknown. One contributor says: "Well over a foot." "I've been stretching on and off for about 29 years. I can wear 11 split collars for a stretch to about eight inches," reports a member of Men_Into_Ball_Stretching. Another stretcher reports to the Everything Ballz Yahoo! group: "I'm stretching my sac with the intent of balls hanging at least 10 inches."

Jarod Johansen, who recently created his website The Art of Ball Stretching, says, "I'm excited to extend a helping hand to those interested in learning how they can gain a lower hanging and larger scrotal sack."

Among the thirty-two sets of five photos each, once sold by Added Dimensions [a California firm that marketed pictures of "horse-hung men from all walks of life"] were two entitled "Men With Bull Balls." A catalogue described one of these sets:

> For many of us, bull balls are a real turn on. These are men who have developed secret techniques for increasing the size of their testicles or lengthening their ballsacs. Jacques, a hot French-Canadian, bends over and shows how far his suckable balls dangle down, and Frank has a set of nuts that hang so low he fits thirteen (count 'em) cock rings around his sac. These nuts hang halfway to his knees. You won't see a photo like this anywhere else.

Not true. A number of comprehensive adult members-only Yahoo! Groups concerned with testicles provide a section of often incredible photos. The Very Lowhangers group home page shows Franky stretching his balls down close to his kneecaps, using a car battery and a roll of lead weighing forty-one pounds. Kindred groups include Balls Lowhanging, Men_Into_Ball_Stretching ( claiming over 4000 members), and Ball Stretching, the latter urging its members to "post photos of your own or other's low hanging balls, both with and without stretching equipment."

One stretcher, "now 52 years old, married for 28 years with three children," provided painstaking details after explaining that he had been inspired "by a photo of an Australian guy who had stretched his scrotum over a foot in length."

Newart Products, an online company, promotes its line of ball stretchers. "Want a pair of low hanging balls? Ever notice how some guys' balls just dangle freely, while others have them tight and almost up inside their bodies? Using ball stretchers over time can help your nuts to hang lower."

The Newart site describes one-, two-, and three-inch leather ball stretchers and split collar stainless steel rings, costing from $30 to $157. It informs the consumer that you can wear multiple rings to stretch to a length that is comfortable for you or increase the number of rings as you gradually lengthen your sack. The rings have two bolts that unscrew.

Have questions? Newart conveniently enables viewers to chat online with a staff member.

Among other stretching devices, the simplest are rings of metal and plastic. One "serious ball stretchers" chat room respondent writes: "I started stretching at six rings. I'm now at 21 rings. I hope when I get to about 8 inches it [the scrotal sack] no longer retracts."

Historians of scrotum-stretching might parenthetically mention that "Testicle Stretch" is the title of an art piece by the American morbid photographer Joel-Peter Witkin and also the name of a track by obscure '80s avant-garde vinyl-mangler Gum.

There is no reference to the use of any stretching device in the nasty but clever Fox sitcom about the life of puppets living in the United States. An old man (actually the puppet Count Blah) talks about his testicles: "Mine hang so low I need a cold shower before I can get on an escalator."

The owner of the Low Hanging Balls 101 website writes that there are probably many reasons why one might want low hanging balls. "From my own experience," he admits, "I find men with low hanging balls are more masculine in appearance and more sexually exciting." He adds, "I also have found that big low hangers are a good way of attracting other men." Also remarking about a pair of pendulous testicles other devotees online refer "to their true beauty," to their being "a huge turn on," and to their giving "a heightened self esteem."

## Tattoos

While some tattoo artists in this country refuse to decorate scrotums, the late premier tattoo artist Roy Boy Cooper of Gary, Indiana told this author long ago that in a single year he had tattooed a couple dozen. Some of these were included in Roy Boy's two videos, *Exotic Expressions* and *Ink Up and Pierce Out*.

Another major figure in the body mod business was the legendary Sailor Sid Diller, a founder of the piercing movement and a famous tattoo artist. Working out of his Silver Anchor studio in Fort Lauderdale, Diller pierced and tattooed exclusively gay men. He informed this author that he had tattooed "quite a number" of scrotums, including his own. One job he especially recalled: tattooing a flame design on a Miami man who had "a terrific set of nuts."

For a fictional instance of tattooed testicles, look no further than novelist Jerry Stahl's wildly careening *Plainclothes Naked* about two crack heads who accidentally steal a photo of nude George W. Bush — a picture revealing a pair of smiley faces tattooed on the family baubles.

The one glittering idea in scrotal adornment is unequivocally a

Swarovski crystal tattoo, or as someone has termed it, "a discoball-esque scrotum." Balldazzling (also called "scrotazzling" or "tea-ba-zzling") is the male equivalent of vajazzling — the act of applying glitter or jewels to a woman's waxed nether regions.

Using your Vajazzle home kit (selling online for as little as $14.95) proceed as follows: (1) shave the area to be decorated and clean the skin; let it dry completely, (2) peel the clear film from the white back-ing (the top of the crystals should stick to the clear film, the bottom of the crystals with the adhesive should be exposed), (3) line up the pattern as you desire, and (4) press firmly and hold for a few seconds.

Your kit will include three crystal tattoo designs of your choice (such as lips, dollar sign, "juicy") and three alcohol wipes to clean the design-selected area. The pattern will last for days, and can be eas-ily removed. The Swarovski crystal tattoos are made in Austria, and resemble diamonds.

Quick instructions on balldazzling at home can be seen on JoeBrener's video, *Ball Dazzling*, on YouTube.

## Inflation

Josey Vogels, in discussing scrotum inflation or infusion on her sex, dating, and relationship website, says the practice involves dip-ping the scrotum in hot wax several times to relax it, injecting a cath-eter into both sides of the balls, and dripping saline solution from an intravenous bag into the scrotum "until your bag looks like a water balloon at a kid's birthday party."

Scrotal inflation supplies include: kit ($22.00), two-hook IV pole ($75.00), solution administration set ($7.50), sterile saline for injec-tion ($9.75) IV catheter ($4.75) and scrotal measuring tape for scrotal potency evaluation ($36.00).

One practitioner says he likes the warm heavy feeling he gets when he's all puffed up. "It feels like I have a fucking ball between my legs! It is the hottest feeling I have ever encountered."

In Catherine Gund Saalfield's riveting 1989 90-minute documentary, *Hallelujah! Ron Athey: A Story of Deliverance*, the performer, provocateur, and pariah offers transfixing rituals that include inflating his testicles to grapefruit size with a saline infusion. This is a movie definitely not for the squeamish or the sexually prudish.

A Miami-area man claimed he had, over an eight-year span, increased the length of his testicles to a prodigious thirteen inches and their circumference to twenty inches through daily vacuum pumping. "I find this [testicle pumping] to be a safe, sensuous, and rewarding hobby," he said. Another man exuberantly offered this testimonial to the Web's Large Penis Support Group: "I wish I'd found pumping a little earlier in life, but here are the results of the last three-and-a-half years: when I started my left testicle was about the size of a small pecan and the right was about twice that size. Three-and-a-half years later the left is the size of a large hen's egg and the right is about twice that size. There are hardly any clothes I can wear that they don't show. Do I care? Nope. I have a lot of fun with it."

The pumping procedure involves placing a tube over the testicles and connecting the attached plastic hose to a manual or electric vacuum pump. Reportedly "results will only come a small amount at a time, over a long period of time — years, not weeks or months — if you pump on a regular basis."

Should you wish to view the method, two sexually explicit videos that include pumping sequences were produced by the now deceased gay superstar Al Parker: *Strange Places, Strange Things* and *High Tech*.

For those wishing how-to-do-it details there's Gary Griffin's manual *The Vacuum Pumper's Handbook*.

Every issue of *BCQ* (Ball Club Quarterly) carried several pages of photographic reproductions — upwards of fifty -- showing scrotums that had been or were being enlarged to grotesque dimensions. In addition, the publication announced the availability of several videos, all having "a completely obsessed theme." Titles included: *Elephant Balls, Aching Balls, Nasty Ball Dreams, Memorable Balls,* and *Friday*

*Night Ball* in which "Mark shows us his unique ability to make his egg size balls dance in their loose sac."

## Other Feats

Then there is the feat never practiced in workout gyms: ball weight lifting. A boot or a bucket gradually being filled with water can be used; a set of metal weights can also work. *BCQ* instructed: "Start light. Work your way up to a plateau of about 15# and then go for more in about 5# increments. Once you get used to the weight itself, try swinging 'em in a geometric pattern. Caution: Do not drop 'em sharply."

An additional stunt was an act that used to take place in a Tokyo bar, until police brought a stop to the performance ... too much noise. A waiter, wearing nothing beneath his short coat, upon serving you your drink would invite you to "watch this." He would pull up his scrotum, insert two matches under the foreskin, proceed to pump a gaseous substance within it, and then light a match. *Abracadabra*: a fire-breathing dragon.

Another exotic diversion involving the scrotum is described graphically by English naval officer William Bligh, who sailed to the Pacific near the end of the eighteenth century. In his first-journey account Bligh recounts a performance by male members of a religious and performing group in pre-Christian Tahiti "which of all things that was ever beheld I imagine was the most uncommon and detestable."

One man — the second of three — brought his stones to the head of his penis and with a small cloth bandage he wrapped them at the same time very violently until they were near a foot in length which the bandage kept them eract at [sic], the stones and the head of the penis being like three small balls at the extremity. The third person was more horrible than the other two, for with both hands seizing the extremity of the scrotum, he pulled it out with such force that the penis went in totally out of sight and the scrotum shockingly distended. In this manner they danced about the ring for a few minutes when I desired them to desist and the Heivah ended. It however afforded much laughter among the spectators.

## Advantageous Clothing

Men who have scrotums of admirable dimensions and an urge to flaunt them might consider Koala "male enhancing" swimwear. The firm's Creation G-string makes use of "a heavy duty elastic band that squeezes your testicles out and forward creating a handsome display." The Jewels Thong is "a beautifully crafted swimsuit that splits and fully exposes your family jewels"; the v-shaped front pouch "plunges deeply between the balls to completely separate and highlight each individually." The Luscious style incorporates a "one-of-a-kind elastic squeeze tunnel." According to Koala's online description, "The Tunnel's for your balls. It firmly glides them out front and exposes them for all to see." The retailer's Diablo Probe "is perfectly balanced with a ball splitter that creates not only a beautiful display but separates and details each testicle for intense pleasure."

# CHAPTER II

# The Pleasures of Feeling and Savoring

In her book *The Nude Male*, Margaret Walters makes numerous references to the penis, but none whatsoever to the testicles. The same goes for Anka Radakovich in *The Wild Girls Club — Tales from Below the Belt*, about "women's little get-togethers where the towel-snapping is held in check but the talk is equally steamy and uninhibited." Radakovich devotes one entire chapter to "A Hard Look at Penises," but doesn't so much as mention the word "scrotum" nor refer to its contents in all 321 pages.

English writer Wayland Young would hardly have applauded the omission. "Bear in mind," he extolled, "that there is in the world such a noble thing as a pair of balls."

John Atkins in his book *Sex in Literature* observes that testicles do not get a very wide literary treatment; he explains: "They do not contribute to the pleasure and tend to be admired on the entirely rational grounds that they are a storehouse of energy."

Not everyone agrees. Cynthia Heimel in her bestseller *Sex Tips For Girls* points out that "The testicles ... enjoy a little licking and fondling also, and become down-right surly if they don't get any." Mindful of this, the authors of *The Clitoral Kiss: A Fun Guide to Oral Sex for*

*Men and Women* lyrically recommend: "Slither around the scrotum with the Snake Tongue. Maybe try Hummin' with the scrotum, half or whole, gently in your mouth. Then play with Gentle Breezes and the Sun Kiss."

With similar scrotal devotion George Krumsback begins his brief encomium "Honor Thy Comrade's Gonads": *Praise be to thee, sac full of seeds of life. Complete with your own implanter. Be a true worshipper. Hang low and humbly before us to solemnly give thanks and worship in sacrificial offering. Amen.* This pietistic tribute appeared in an issue of the pre-Web era *Ball Club Quarterly*, "a communications network for men who have 'em and men who want 'em." The fellowship, founded in Pomona, California in 1985, claimed more than 400 fetishistic members, not only in the United States but in Europe and Australia as well. Like most other periodicals aimed at a gay readership, *BCQ* carried columns and columns of that "odd and compact art form," the personal ad. In fact, half of each 76-page issue — "There are virtually no limits to the kinds of activities that you may seek or find through the pages of *BCQ*" — was devoted to such communications.

These days, such messaging is fast and free via the Internet. Every website testicles group with a mainly or exclusively gay membership provides chances to forward messages, such as:

Love to suck those gonads
Gonads, what I love to lick
Take each one into my mouth
While I stroke his dick

## Sucking: Desire and Techniques

"I think my boyfriend wants me to suck his balls. I've never heard of this. Do you have any advice?" queries a *Cosmopolitan* reader of Amy Levine, Cosmo's Carnal Counselor. To which the advisor gives this elaborately instructive reply:

Your guy's request is far from unusual. Sucking on his testicles can make for an incredibly sensational experience.

Next time you're giving him south-of-the border oral action, take a sexy detour and move your mouth from his main member to the rest of his package. Swirl the tip of your tongue around his scrotum — the loose sac of skin that surrounds the testicles. Then, lick his balls with long, sweeping strokes as if you were savoring a delicious ice cream cone.

Mix it up and intermittently purse your lips and suck softly on the skin or take each testicle all the way into your mouth.

Acclaimed contemporary American novelist Anne Rice, widely popular for her *Interview with the Vampire* and its sequel *The Vampire Lestat* as well as *Cry to Heaven* and *The Feast of All Saints*, and creator of the rather racy literary alter ego A.N. Roquelaure, clearly knows a thing or two (or three) about pampering testicles. In *Beauty's Punishment*, [book two of Rice's trilogy of Roquelaure books that is a "bare-assed parody" of the Sleeping Beauty fairy tale], we read, in contrast to earlier strictly sadistic passages, the following description by the "tall, heavily muscled" Prince Tristan, the "disobedient slave":

My tongue lapped at the soft, salty skin [of a powerfully built blond-haired slave — one of several princes] lifting the balls and letting them slide out of my mouth, then lapping fast again, trying to cover them, as the taste of the warm flesh and salt intoxicated me. The Prince wriggled and danced as I licked, his extraordinarily muscled legs flexing up and down as much as the space would allow. I mouthed all the scrotum sucking on it, nipping at it.

Later on we're told about another sensual moment:

He urged me back gently and with his left hand he lifted his balls and his cock. I dropped down and kissed his balls immediately. I ran my tongue over them as I had been taught to do with the ponies in the stable, mouthing them and feeling them tenderly with my teeth.

To induce similar attention from his own wife, Tommy Lee, celebrated drummer for the Mötley Crüe rock band, once was said to be thinking about having his testes message tattooed: *Suck Here, This ball's for you*, and *fondle us*.

Real-life specifics are provided by the Society for Human Sexuality on its Web page "The Art of Oral Sex ":

Don't forget his balls; it can be fun for both of you if you play them right. Begin by gently licking his balls with your tongue. You may want to gently caress his cock with your hand while you're bathing his balls with your tongue. Remember that the balls are sensitive to excessive pressure. However, it can feel good to him if you put your thumb and forefinger around his sack and pull on it surprisingly hard in fact.

Once you get them wet try taking one of them into your mouth and playing with it; see if you can get both of them in. Watch his face, and feel him quivering as you gently move them around in your mouth.

When Topix.com asked, "How do you treat the balls during sex?" 43% replied, "fondle/caress 'em"; 29% "suck 'em"; and 10% "lick'em."

Go Ask Alice!, a health question and answer Internet resource, in talking about ball-sucking says that "sucking and tongue action can be combined with hot breaths, as well as blowing cool streams of air." She likens ball-sucking to "eating a lollipop."

# Teabagging

A related practice, "the hot new sexual act," is descriptively called "teabagging" — lowering one's scrotum into another person's mouth in the fashion of a teabag into a mug, with an up/down motion. The term appeared in an episode of the television series *Sex and the City* when Samantha Jones explained the act quite blatantly and loudly in a crowded restaurant. It gained national attention again in the DVD version of the open-road adventure *Jay and Silent Bob Strike Back* when Jay sings "teabag my balls."

" ... and a lollipop man started teabagging you" is a line from the "First Kiss" routine by the three-piece British sitcom group We Are Klang. The bawdy stunt again was mentioned in the animated TV series *Family Guy* when Stewie Griffin asks if Dylan would like to teabag him at his naked tea party.

The nationally distributed 1998 "ebulliently trashy" film *Pecker* [available on DVD] directed by John Waters [*Serial Mom, Hairspray*] includes a show-stopping phenomenon. At a Baltimore gay bar dubbed the Fudge Palace, the director introduces the practice in which rough-trade go-go dancers "dangle and dunk their balls onto fat, bold patrons' foreheads."

AskMen.com advisor Donald Zimmer suggests "you can always have her [him] lie down and place your testes softly in her [his] mouth." Ballsuction, a Yahoo! adult group having over 3400 members as of 2012, provides, according to its home page, "clips of one of the more pleasant things a girl can do to her guy: suctioning his balls with her mouth." At least a half dozen other Yahoo! groups include teabagging as a major interest.

Totally Tasteless studio has produced a series of five *Teabaggers* DVDs: "Get your sweaty balls out and swinging 'cause these girls love chugging on hanging nuts! It's a jolly teabaggin' time for all, so come in and join the fun," invites one promotion.

Website Photobucket ("the place to store, create, and share your photos for life") provides over 200 teabagging pictures, including one showing the cover of the fanciful *Teabagging for DUMMIES*.

The online Lovers' Guide ["The world's no. 1 for sex and relation-ships"] refers to teabagging as "a neat variation on oral sex, allowing you to take what might be a much needed break from sucking his penis."

"They [the testes] certainly do contribute to pleasure; ... more so because they are in the pelvic region," emphasized William Young, when director of clinical services for the former world-famous Masters and Johnson Institute in St. Louis. He added that there is a lot happen-ing in the testes prior to ejaculation, providing enjoyable sensations beyond that of touch.

Website JackinWorld's fifth anniversary in 2002 asked readers to "Please rate the following parts of your body by how sensitive they are to erotic touch." Regarding the scrotum, of the 5005 responses 44.1% indicated "very sensitive," 42.0% "somewhat sensitive."

## Fondling

Descriptions of torrid reveries in some sexually oriented periodi-cals occasionally include references to the testicles. Those in *Playgirl*'s monthly fantasies feature: "I ... reached farther down to feel his balls. That really drove him crazy." "I reached for his balls and slowly ca-ressed and squeezed them." "I traced the path of the vein with my tongue and teeth nipping at the curly hair rising around the base, my hands softly cupping and massaging his balls. One at a time I gently sucked his balls into my mouth and slowly rolled them across my tongue." " ... her fingers sought out my jewel-bags, kneading and caressing them like rolls of warm sensuous dough."

Related material appears in dirty jokes, male braggadocio, fe-male gossip, bawdy song, and erotic novels. Among the latter, turn to the first and arguably the best book of pornography in the English language: John Cleland's *Memoirs of a Woman of Pleasure* [later re-named *Fanny Hill* when rewritten] legally available in the US only since 1963, and in England since 1970. Privately printed in 1748-49, it is structured in the form of a series of first-person letters addressed to an unnamed "Madam," wherein Fanny sets out to confess all the "scandalous stages of my life." She journeys to the big city, she falls in love, she needs money to live on, her lovers have careers and positions, and in the end, settling into middle-class respectability, she marries the man of her choice.

The Bishop of London blamed the book for two minor London earthquakes and called it "an open insult upon Religion and Good manners, and a reproach to the Honour of government and the Law of Country."

For a book of this nature, Cleland's prose is remarkable and refreshing. He employs no obscene or objectionable words; instead he proved himself "a master of the sexual metaphor." Early in her account Fanny admits she "admired ... the roundish bag that dangled" from one of her lovers. Later in her description of one Charles, with whom she lodged for a while, she refers to his "globular appendage, the wondrous treasure bag of nature's sweets, which lay revealed round, and pursed up in the only wrinkles that are known to please ...." Fanny goes on to relate:

> Presently he guided my hand lower to that part in which nature and pleasure keep their stores in concert, so aptly  fastened and hung onto the root of their first instrument ... that might not improperly be styled their purse bearer  too; there he made me feel distinctly through their cover the contents, a pair of roundish balls that seemed to play within, and elude all pressure, but the tenderest from without."

Further on Fanny writes about Will, "my new humble sweetheart," describing his "bottom appendage, the unsurpassed purse of ladies' jewels ...." Later she confides that she stole her hand softly "to that store bag of nature's sweets which is attached to its conduit pipe from which we receive them."

In describing another playmate, Fanny again metaphorically writes about the "rich appendage of the treasure bag beneath, large in proportion ...."

About a century and a half following the publication of Cleland's book, the infamous *My Secret Life — the Sex Diary of a Victorian Gentleman* came out in Amsterdam. Banned in England for the next hundred years for being obscene and pornographic, the eleven-volume work was picked by *Time Out* in 2008 as one of London's "30 finest-ever-peddlers of smut, filth, and depravity." The anonymous author [believed to be one Henry Spencer Ashbee] makes 12 references to the scrotum, 29 to testicles, 69 to bullock, and 110 to balls. For instance: "Sophy would handle my balls gently at first, then squeeze one stone, then the other, then hold the bag in her fist. Her language also had a ballocky tone — 'Let's feel your balls — how's your bolly?'" Later on: "The way she nestled her nose round my balls was curious — most women have a way of their own in amorous tricks."

A couple hundred years before Cleland's legendary *Memoirs,* the notorious "scourge of princes," Pietro Aretino, produced the first erotic book in the Christian world to be written in the vulgar tongue of ordinary speech. He also wrote poetry and plays and theological works, lives of the saints, and lampoons on the living, and nearly became a cardinal.

"Whore dialogues," a literary genre of the Renaissance and the Enlightenment and a type of erotic fiction, typically concerned the sexual education of a naïve younger woman and an experienced older woman. In Aretino's satiric *Dialogo nel quale la Nanna insegna a la Pippa* (1536) of grotesque wit, Nanna vividly relates her sexual experiences during her years as a nun and later as a courtesan. To Pippa, her daughter: "Pippa, though I tell people you are only sixteen, the truth is that you are twenty, round and clear, since you were born just before the opening of Leo's conclave. When all over Rome you could hear them crying: 'Balls! Balls!' I was groaning 'Oh God help me!' In fact, I made you just when they were hanging the Medici ball-bedecked coat-of-arms over the gate of St. Peter's."

Later, in giving Pippa instructions in "the art of being a whore," Nanna says: "There's not a single man who does not touch heaven with his finger when the girl he is making love to, while slipping her tongue into the side of his mouth, grabs his rod ... then, after waiting a while, she takes his balls in the palm of her hand and starts scratching them tenderly." Again in enlightening Pippa, Nanna confides: "what a murderous job it is for a women working at pleasure to get a man who wants to have his balls scratched and tickled."

Such pampering is recommended by Eva Margolies in her primer on men's sexual problems and what women can do to help them.

She advises women to examine the scrotum: "Feel the skin on the scrotal sac, and note how similar it feels to your own inner vaginal lips." Then urges Margolies: "Don't forget to ask if and how he enjoys having his testicles fondled."

In the hilarious book *Sex Tips for Straight Women from a Gay Man* ("Who knows more about what men like than a gay man?") the authors write delicately: "We believe that balls have always been treated like unwelcome country cousins. You recognize them when they show up at the door, but you're not so happy to see them, because you have absolutely no idea of what would keep them entertained." You can kiss confusion goodbye after reading the Play Ball chapter.

The Society for Human Sexuality's Internet "Lesson Nine" of the fourteen-lesson tutorial on fellatio declares: "You will discover an entirely new world of sensations for your partner when you take time to get to know his testicles."

In the lesson "How to Give the Perfect Hand Job," instructor Peter Brooks recommends: " ... slip your hand down his testicles and ever so gently grab them in your fingers, softly tugging them down away from his shaft. If they are big and bulky like grade AA eggs, bounce them up the underside of his shaft. He will like the way this feels."

*Redbook* Web page "35 Sexy New Places to Touch Your Man" lists "The scrotal sac" and "The male G-spot": "Gently roll his testicles in your palm. Fiddle with the hardened seminal vesicles. This will drive him nearly mad."

*Redbook* online offers additional tantalizing specifics in "5000 Men Reveal Their Other Hot Spots":

> Imagine if your husband slipped a silk scarf between your legs with such a light touch you weren't sure you actually felt something, except that you most definitely knew you wanted more. That's the kind of subtly exquisite feeling you can elicit from a man by handling his prized possessions with tender loving care. As long as you don't pinch, squeeze, or dig in your nails, all you need worry about is how much pleasure your man can take. He'll love it if you lightly scratch his testicles and gently pull or rub his scrotum. If you want to turn up the sexual volume, try caressing him wearing satin gloves or sneaking undercover to stake out the new territory with your mouth and tongue.

Elsewhere about "12 Amazing Tricks He Secretly Wants You to Know" *Redbook's* Dr. Ava Cadell writes: " ... testicles can be touched and, boy, should they be touched. Pinch, tug, suck on his testicles. Linger. Dawdle. Don't make this an after-thought. This is a destination in itself."

From Britain, that "urban jungle of emerging sexuality," comes this advice: "Give your man something truly special," implores Marsha Ann Folks, who then details: "Tell him to close his eyes and prepare for a surprise. Take one testicle in each hand and quickly squeeze as hard as you can. Don't worry, you can't hurt him. Actually the most common mistake is of forcing the semen out and triggering an immediate incredibly powerful orgasm." Folks continues: "It is not uncommon for men to groan, writhe, flail, or even scream at this point. Keep squeezing for 10-20 seconds until he calms down and his whole body relaxes. Then let go." The bottom line: "He'll remember you for the rest of his life."

Some sexologists call attention to the scrotal seam, which has more passion-packing ability than you might have thought. Online Love & Sex Shopping Lifestyle points out that the raphe [the strong dividing line between the left and right halves of the scrotal sac] is a particular spot that can "literally send him into orbit when touched." It adds: "Turns out, this is a major moan zone for guys."

The raphe (pronounced RAY-fee) can be stimulated by gently running your fingertips along it," instructs Yvonne K. Fulbright, popular television personality, advice columnist, and author of the erotic and playful manual *Touch Me There! — a Hands-On Guide to Your Orgasmic Hot Spots* (2007).

Some men love having their R-spot stimulated, while others find it too intense. If your guy digs it, try running the top of your tongue along the area, flicking the seam while still toying with his boys with your hands.

The raphe marks the position of the scrotal septum, a wall of connective tissue inside that separates the scrotum into two halves, each of which contains a testis.

## Massaging

Supposedly more medical than erotic is the so-called ancient Thai style of testicle massage. A one-and-a-half hour "sexually stimulating" treatment that includes manipulation of the testes by a Dream Teen hostess in Pattaya, Thailand will cost $20.00 [700 baht].

One customer described his experience in detail:

With a pumping action she massaged the area surrounding my testicles, but not the testicles directly. Using her thumb and fingers she massaged at the base, pulling down as she massaged. She did this for about five minutes after which she gripped my balls at the root and lightly pulled them down, up, then down again, continually. Lightly applying pressure to my testicles, she massaged all around them, working her way around one then the other then both of them. She stretched out my testicle skin until it felt loose and comfortable. Methodically grasping around the base of my testicles with her thumb and forefinger she squeezed until they were tight, and then positioned them on top of her fingers. With her other hand she then applied a small amount of pressure on top of the testicles and massaged them in a circular motion. While she was doing this she also pulled down lightly on the hand grabbing the base of my testicles' connecting flesh. It took about ten minutes and afterwards my testicles felt unbelievable.

The tourist concluded with this suggestion: "If you've been neglecting your balls all these years like I have, take them on a holiday to Thailand."

An article "dedicated to women's sexuality" offers these instructions for massaging the testicles:

First take hold of the scrotum with your whole hand, warming it inside your hand, and massaging it gently by gripping movements. Warming and handling the scrotum gives feelings in the whole genital region. The testicles are best stimulated by gently rolling movements with your fingers. Also tickle the scrotal skin with your finger tips.

A reader asks Sue of the PassionVillage website: "I heard about a simple trick where if one squeezes the testicles it prevents premature ejaculation from happening as quickly." To which Sue replies: "There is a technique used to prevent premature ejaculation that's more of a testicle pull than a squeeze, but women have been using it for centuries to slow down men who are a 'little quick off the mark.' Here's the deal: Just before a man ejaculates his testicles move up against his body. If you gently hold down his scrotum and prevent his lift he is unable to ejaculate." She adds, "Catherine the Great apparently tied silk scarves around the testicles of her lovers to prevent any type of ejaculation, and had them beheaded if they didn't perform."

More deviant still: To satisfy his insatiable craving for scrotal attention, not long ago in Sidney, Australia Craig Bell, a 43-year-old banker, by design had his scrotum checked over more than 300 times, mainly by female doctors. He would visit local clinics to get examined by complaining about having been hit in the groin with a bat or ball. One doctor told the court that after the odeous happening she had difficulty examining other male patients. Bell was sentenced to 240 hours of community service on 24 counts of sexual assault.

## Toys

Among the unending variety of sex toys available online and from sex and novelty shops is the Rocco Series Venetian, designed to promote and maintain an erection while stimulating the testicles and clitoris. According to an item in *Playgirl*: "By slipping the rubber contraption over your honey's hotdog, as you would a ring on a finger, and placing the Jel-lee balls against his own, you'll delight in hours of rock-hard entertainment — replete with gasps and moans."

Two additional heterosexual devices are the Diving Dolphin and the Adonis Pouch. The former has separate vibrators to stimulate the clitoris and testicles simultaneously. "Start revving your engine," says an ad, "there's going to be orgasm all around with this one." The Pouch is a multi-speed stimulator that massages the testicles. According to an ad, the penis support ring encourages "long-lasting hard-ons while the vibration provides clitoral stimulation for your partner."

Then there's an "ultra-realistic dill for those who want it all including the testicles" of high-density silicone, distributed by Womyn's Ware, Inc. According to the Canadian company's Web page: "Some women find that when these toys are worn in a harness they can place the testicles low over the clit for extra stimulation." The Johnny dill's testicles come complete with a skin-like wrinkled texture ("one slightly larger than the other, of course."). Color choice: black and vanilla. Price: $99.85. The company's catalogue also shows the Package dildo (caramel color only),which has "testicles so realistic you almost expect them to squeal when you squeeze them."

One testicular device you won't find in any shops or sex toy catalogues is the *godemiché* — a refined velvet or glass innovation at one time used in France. Achieving tremendous popularity in the eighteenth century, it was an artificial scrotum that could be filled with hot milk. Compressing this little sack was intended to simulate ejaculation. Such was among those apparatuses used by women to excite their *libido sexualis*.

# CHAPTER III

# A Diversion: A Testicular Miscellany

What makes a man? We may never know. But scientists now think they do know what makes a male masculine.

They have found a key gene on the Y chromosome that seems to act as a "master switch for maleness," transforming a growing human fetus, which otherwise would become a girl, into a baby boy.

During the seventh week of pregnancy, the gene sets off a bio-chemical cascade that turns the fetus's immature sex organs into testes. Without this genetic activity, the budding sex organs would develop into ovaries.

These glands, within a couple of months before or just after birth, drop into the loose, multi-layered pouch of skin called the scrotum [a medieval perversion of *scortum*, meaning skin or hide], which serves mainly to house and protect them. This departure of the testis is a strange, complex, and incompletely understood phenomenon that occurs only in certain mammals. In man it brings the testes into a realm of lower temperature, essential for the maturation of sperms. In whales, elephants, and some others whose body temperature is lower than in man, the testes are tucked up in the relative safety of the ab-dominal cavity, while in rats and bats they descend only during the breeding season, then withdraw until the next cycle.

The testicles of the young squirrel-like tree shrew from Southeast

Asia remain in the body as long as the animal is in a stressful environment. But about a week after it is moved to serene surroundings, the testicles will enter the scrotum. When the adult animal is being disturbed, the testicles will move back into the abdominal cavity, their weight will decrease, and sperm production will cease.

It is possible for human males to draw the testes up for protection. One of the first lessons in Chinese methods of boxing is to train the cremaster [the muscles by which the testicles are suspended] to withdraw the testes from harm.

The free-hanging scrotum and testes in most of the higher primates are obviously vulnerable, but "apparently this factor is of overriding importance only in the gibbon, which swings through the trees with folded legs, and whose testes are held close to the body wall and cannot be observed."

Entomologist Robert L. Smith attracted considerable notice in 1984 when he suggested that the external location of testicles has to do with "sperm competition." He theorized that promiscuous species have testicles on the outside because their sperm must be kept cool and "in fighting trim" in order to compete with the sperm of other males when deposited in the females' reproductive tracts.

Another explanation can be deduced from a theory of evolution formulated ten years earlier than Smith's speculations by Israeli evolutionary biologist Amotz Zahavi: Men have pendulous testicles because women want it that way.

The dawn of precise understanding of the structure and function of these glands came with John Hunter, the eighteenth-century British anatomist. During the same period, several monographs on the testis by French and English surgeons appeared: notably Sir Astley Paston Cooper's *Observations on the Structure and Diseases of the Testes* (1830) and Thomas Blizard Curling's 568-page book *A Practical Treatise on Diseases of the Testicle, Spermatic Cord, and Scrotum*, which went through four editions between 1843 and 1878 and was translated into French and Chinese.

From clinical examination and post-mortem dissection a comprehensive picture of the testicles emerged: Within each one there are about 250 compartments, each of which contains one to three small tightly coiled tubes one to two feet long, the aggregate length totaling several hundred yards. The walls of these tubes are lined with germinal tissue, and it is here that the development of sperm — the process known as spermatogenesis — takes place. These tubes, some 600 to 1200 of them, meet at a core-like structure (the rete testis), a network of vessels in the upper portion of the testicle. This meshwork of tubes, fibers, and vessels empties into ten to fifteen ducts (vasa efferentia), through which the sperm — the smallest cells in the body — are moved by successive waves of contractions to the epididymis, a fifty-foot duct tightly coiled in each testicle. It is in this chamber of maturation that the sperm remain to ripen for as long as seventy-two days before the eight-to-ten-day journey ahead.

Each testicle is suspended from its compartment by a spermatic cord. Often the left cord is the longer. Concerning this, a 1975 study noted that in right-handed men the right testis tended to be higher, and surprisingly the heavier and of greater volume.

The author, an anonymous "French army surgeon" according to the title page, of a nineteenth-century book "strictly limited to One Thousand numbered copies" in discussing suspension of the testicles mentions that "The younger and more vigorous the man from a genital point of view, the nearer are the testicles drawn to the top of the purses ...." In an old man, he writes, the testicle loses its oblique position to assume a nearly horizontal position across the purses, which become elongated. He adds: "A similar disposition is also to be remarked in young men who have indulged too freely in venereal pleasures. We have even remarked it in a young man of 17, exhausted by masturbation."

Testicles manufacture the spermatozoa (a name coined in 1827) needed to perpetuate the race: an estimated 85 to 115 million cells a day. In fact, every two months enough seeds are produced in a single male theoretically to populate the entire earth. They also produce the hormone of maleness, testosterone, a secretion that influences physical growth and psychic development. The hormone, first isolated nearly half a century ago, is responsible for development and preservation of facial and body hairs, muscular and skeletal development, and attraction to the opposite sex. It also controls the development, size, and function of the seminal vesicles (small sacs), prostate, penis, and scrotum.

Its main effects, though, according to noted neuroanatomist Dr. Norman Geschwind at Harvard Medical School and his colleague Dr. Albert Galaburda, are in the areas of the brain that control speech, spatial abilities, and handedness. Its influence on behavior remains largely a matter of creative speculation. The commonly held belief that testosterone produces antisocial behavior may be a misconception. Researchers are now finding that high levels make men energetic, friendly, easy-going, and sexy, "rather like a Teddy Pendergrass CD."

Testosterone levels in the fetus can vary with such factors as the amount of psychological stress the mother feels, maternal diet, and possibly even the season of the year.

Curiously, this chemical of manhood is also found in women, but it is only one-twentieth the amount found in men. Without it, a woman could be frigid, and with an oversupply, masculinized.

The activities of the testicles were unknown to the ancients. In fact, the origin of spermatozoa in the testes, and their function, were disputed until the early nineteenth century.

The mythology before ancient Greece treated procreation as a purely feminine function. The Hippocratic treatise *On Semen* recognized a female seed, and centuries later the Greek physician Galen argued that the "female testes," or ovaries — one on each side of the uterus — produced a true sperm that had the power of generation after being mixed with the male seminal fluid. To Galen, the only difference between a male's testes and those of a female was that the male's are contained in a scrotum.

Several centuries later, in the mid-1500s, Renaldus Columbus wrote: "Testes are produced in women so that they may produce semen. Indeed I myself can bear witness that, in the dissection of female testicles, I have sometimes found semen ... as all the spectators have acknowledged with one voice."

Albertus Magnus, the thirteenth-century German theologian, writer, scientist, and scholastic philosopher, known as the Universal Doctor, wrote that "we must accept that generation materially is from what is called women's sperm ...."

In the fifteenth century, Leonardo da Vinci reasoned that sperm is formed in the testicles, since a male whose testicles are removed is made sterile. He concluded that "the testicles increase the animosity and ferocity of animals. The principle is clearly illustrated in the case of castrated animals, for one sees the bull, the boar, the ram, and the cock, very fierce animals, which after having been deprived of these testicles remain very cowardly ...."

But Leonardo's studies had little effect on contemporary scientists. Aristotle was aware that the testes were essential for the virility and fertility of male animals; but by not recognizing the testes of serpents or fishes, he decided they "are merely attached [to the ducts] just like the stone weights which women hang on their looms when they are weaving." This belief that the testes served merely to keep the attached vas deferens, or seminal duct, straight and unkinked would seem to explain the vernacular reference to "stones."

Among the characteristics of the testes is their mobility. They are the only visible organ of the body that can disappear entirely and involuntarily and cannot be made to reappear voluntarily. This retraction is produced by various conditions: cold, anxiety, closure of the anal sphincter, and sexual arousal. A *Playgirl* magazine reader writing to the periodical's sex advisor, Lolita Sapriel, requested an explanation. She wrote that her husband's "balls rise up into the stomach area as he is coming during sex .... I have noticed that if I masturbate him his balls stay in place if no pressure is on the penis. But if I apply pressure by lifting the penis up, the balls start to rise."

Replied Sapriel: "In the same way that women have uterine contractions during their orgasms, men's testes contract just prior to and during orgasm. Some men have stronger and more noticeable contractions than others ... but it is a normal response." She added: "Since it gives him pleasure and no pain — don't worry about it. He's okay."

A remarkable feature of the scrotum is its regenerative capability. Within a few weeks there can be a complete replacement following loss due to injury or disease. This was well-demonstrated in a case reported in *Medical Aspects of Human Sexuality*. The front of a young man's pants were caught in the rotating power takeoff of a farm tractor. There was nearly a complete tearing away of the skin of the scrotum, which eventually reformed.

According to one estimate, one in every 30 boys under 14 years of age and one in every 250 men over 21 are affected by *cryptorchidism* — an anomaly in which one or both testicles fail to descend. The condition figures in Freud's fascinating account of the Rat Man. The latter had one undescended testicle, with which he was quite often preoccupied and for which he considered his father responsible.

More astonishing is the story of Erika Schinegger, a top Austrian girl skier and winner of the 1966 world downhill title. Erika — now Erik Schinegger — had undescended testicles. Before withdrawing from the national team, the ski champion had been one of Austria's big hopes for a women's medal in the 1968 Olympics. Reportedly, an Olympic staff member had declared: "Whatever he calls himself, there is a man skiing in the Austrian ladies' team."

A reverse of cryptorchidism is the retraction of one or both testicles into the groin or abdominal areas. This is the problem Alexander Portnoy describes at length in Philip Roth's controversial masterpiece novel *Portnoy's Complaint*:

Sometime during my ninth year one of my testicles apparently decided it had had enough of life down in the scrotum and began to make its way north. At the beginning I could feel it as though its moment of indecision has [sic] passed, entering the cavity of my body, like a survivor being dragged up out of the sea and over the hull of a lifeboat. And there it nestled, foolhardy mate, to chance it alone in that boy's world of football cleats and picket fences, sticks and stones and pocket knives, all those dangers that drove my mother wild with foreboding, and about which I was warned and warned and warned. And warned again. And again.

And again.

So my left testicle took up residence in the vicinity of the inguinal canal. By pressing a finger in the crease between my groin and my thigh, I could still, in the early weeks of its disappearance, feel the curve of its jellied roundness; but then came nights of terror, when I searched my guts in vain, searched all the way up to my rib cage — alas, the voyager had struck off for regions uncharted and unknown. Where was it gone to! How high and how far before the journey would come to an end! Would I one day open my mouth to speak in class, only to discover my left nut out on the end of my tongue? In school we chanted, along with our teacher, *I am the Captain of my fate, I am the Master of my soul* and meanwhile, within my own body, an anarchic insurrection had been launched by one of my privates — which I was helpless to put down!

For some six months, until its absence was observed by the family doctor during my annual physical examination, I pondered my mystery, more than once wondering — for there was no possibility that did not enter my head, *none* — if the testicle could have taken a dive backwards toward the bowl and there begun to convert itself into just such an egg as I observed my mother yank in a moist yellow cluster from the dark interior of a chicken whose guts was emptying into the garbage. What if breasts began to grow on me, too! What if my penis went dry and brittle, and one day, while I was urinating, snapped off in my hand? Was I being transformed into a girl? Or worse, into a boy such as I understood (from the playground grapevine) that Robert Ripley of *Believe it or Not* would pay "a reward" of a hundred thousand dollars for? Believe it or not, there is a nine-year-old boy in New Jersey who is a boy in every way, *except he can have babies.*

Who gets the reward? Me, or the person who turns me in?

Doctor Izzie rolled the scrotal sac between his fingers as though it were the material of a suit he was considering buying, and then told my father that I would have to be given a series of male hormone shots. One of my testicles had never fully descended — unusual, not unheard of .... But if the shots don't work, asks my father in alarm. What then — ! Here I am sent out into the waiting room to look at a magazine.

The shots work. I am spared the knife. (Once again!)

Another testicular aberration is monorchism, the condition in which only one testis is apparent, the other being absent or undescended. Since the lone testicle produces sufficient amounts of hormones and sperm for normal physiological and sexual functioning, monorchism is of no clinical significance. It is said that the outstanding Roman general and dictator Sulla (138-78 B.C.) and Tamerlane (1336?-1405), the great Mongol emperor who conquered Persia and Central Asia, were monorchids — reassurances that this abnormality in no way limits a man's ability to perform manly feats. Nevertheless, as Jeremy Taylor points out in his listing of "10 Famous Men With Only One Ball," having a single, lonely nut can be a source of great embarrassment for a guy. It was even worse at one time in France. For a considerable part of the the sixteenth century men who possessed only one testicle were subject to discrimination.

In the next century, on January 5, 1607 to be exact, the High Court of Paris submitted on appeal a verdict in favor of one Claudine Godefroy "that there was just cause that she do not forego the celebration of her nuptials, since the doctors and surgeons affirmed in their report that the man had but one testicle, though they added that he was notwithstanding capable of engendering."

Nonetheless, the belief that both testicles were indispensible for fecundity had prevailed in the *Shulchan 'Aruch*, the legal code of Jewish religious law, and in the edict of Pope Sixtus V (1585-1590) that provided for the dissolution of marriages of men not possessing two testicles. Decades later, Jacopo Caranta, doctor of medicine and philosophy, discussed in his treatise, *De noto cum uno testiculo* ... (1624), whether a man born with only one testicle — or without any — could have sexual intercourse and generate.

It is conjectured that Hitler was a monorchid. The Russian doctors who reportedly performed an autopsy on his body in May 1945 announced: "The left testicle could not be found either in the scrotum or on the spermatic cord inside the inguinal canal, nor in the small pelvis."

None of Hitler's doctors mentions monorchism. Nonetheless, Walter C. Langer in *The Mind of Adolf Hitler* notes how closely Hitler's behavior resembled that of prepubertal boys with a history of behavioral disturbances combined with a missing testicle. And Robert G. L. Waite, author of *The Psychopathic God: Adolph Hitler*, concludes that the Führer acted very much like certain kinds of neurotic monorchids.

Hitler's probable monorchism was exploited by stand-up comic George Carlin noted for his black humor: "You realize Hitler had one ball?" he said to his audiences. "What do you think about a man with one ball? You think he has two strikes against him? Maybe he's got one ball and two strikes. Hitler only had one ball. A lot of people don't know that. A lot of people don't know it. They say, 'Gee, Hitler had a lot of balls.' One."

Then there are the following lines set to the tune "Colonel Bogey March" sung by World War II Tommies:

Hitler has only got one ball.
Göring has two but rather small
Himmler is somewhat sim'lar.
But poor old Goebbels 'as no balls at all!

No balls at all: an anomaly due to one of two causes: (1) *anorchia*, resulting in the absence of both testes at birth, and (2) *castration*, the surgical removal of the sex gland for religious, medical, or social reasons.

*Anorchidism* affects one out of about every 20,000 males at birth. It's the theme of the ditzy folk ditty "No Balls at All":

Oh, come all ye lad-dies and listen to me,
And I'll tell you a tale that will fill you with glee
Of a pretty young maiden so fair and so tall,
Who married a man who had no balls at all!
No balls at all; she married a man who had no balls at all!

The night of the wedding she crept into bed;
Her cheeks were so rosy, her ass was so red.
She reached for his penis, his penis was small;
She reached for his balls, but he'd no balls at all!

"Oh, Mother! Oh, Mother! Oh, what shall I do?
I've married a man who's unable to screw.

My troubles are many, my pleasures are small,
For I've married a man who has no balls at all!"

"Oh, daughter! Oh, daughter! Do not be sad;
The same thing was true when I married your dad.
But there's always a good man awaiting the call
Of the wife of the man who had no balls at all!"

This very wise daughter took mother's advice;
She got herself laid by a man who seemed nice.
And a queer looking bastard was born in the fall,
To the wife of the man who had no balls at all!

The husband was joyous; got high as a kite;
The sight of that infant filled him with delight!
Though its head was too large, and its body too small
The great thing about him — he'd no balls at all!

One can't estimate how many modern-day eunuchs there are in the United States. One of them, a Seattle resident, who fantasized about being castrated most of his life, admits: "I feel very glad to have had my balls cut off." Says another "nutless wonder": "A lot of guys get turned on by the fact that I'm a eunuch — just the idea that I don't have any balls and like to have sex." For anyone enticed by the subject, there's the paperback *The Advantages of Castration* [limited. availability] by Victor T. Cheney.

From "no balls at all" let's turn attention to men who have three or more.

Although you most likely aren't one of them or know someone who is, there are males who possess three testicles. Indeed, triorchidism [also called tritestes] exists in fact and in fiction. And in flights of fancy. One recently published book available from Amazon attempts to answer the question: "What does it mean to dream of three testicles?"

Another query: "Does having three balls improve sex?" One man answers, "Nah, the third one's a little guy; he kinda just hangs in the wings but is fully operational. He's my backup plan." Another replies, "Never had one afraid of mine; he gets mad love." And another: "Man, just wear tight jeans; you'll score with the ladies." "Now if ya had two shlongs, we would be talking," says still another.

Ask someone about the condition and you might possibly get an answer such as the following: "My husband has three testicles — two small ones in one scrotum and a normal size in the other." "My boyfriend just noticed recently that he had a third testicle." "I, too, have three testicles; it is an interesting conversation piece when the time is right."

It's said the males of the renowned Medici family of Florentine bankers, who became rulers of Tuscany, were generously endowed by nature. Generously indeed, if we can speculate about their family crest, which displayed anywhere from six to twelve balls on a gold shield. Declared a contemporary of Cosimo I de' Medici: "He has emblazoned even the monks' privies with his balls."

Commenting on a related Italian Renaissance matter, historian Robert Melville offers this observation about Andrea del Verrocchio's magnificent equestrian statue in Venice of the triumphant captain of the Venetian armies, Bartolomeo Colleoni, [an exact reproduction of which is in Newark, New Jersey]: "As a study of excessive masculinity it lends credence to the rumour, likely to last as long as the effigy itself, that the subject, the condottiere Colleoni, had three testicles." (It is much more likely he had just a hydrocele — a fluid-filled sac surrounding a testicle.) In fact, "Once you know to look for testicles at Colleoni's place, you see them everywhere. Even festooning his tomb. A trio of testicles following you into death. Trailing you through the afterlife."

In the seventeenth century, Gerardus Blasius in his *Observationes medicae rariores* remarked about cases of more than three testicles, and a certain doctor in the nineteenth century named Russell, "one of the older writers on the testicle," in an Edinburgh medical journal item referred to four, five, and even six testicles in one individual: four testes were of usual size; two were smaller.

Then, too, the nineteenth-century *Encyclopedia Collection of Rare and Extraordinary Cases and of the Most Striking Instances of Abnormality in all Branches of Medicine and Surgery, Derived from an Exhaustive Research of Medical Literature from its Origin to the Present* discusses instances of polyorchids — males having three or more testicles. It tells of a monk who was a triorchid "and was so salacious that his indomitable passion prevented him from keeping his vows of chastity." The authors added: "The amorous propensities and generative faculties of polyorchids have always been supposed greater than ordinary." They tell of another man so endowed who was prescribed a concubine "as a reasonable allowance."

The anonymous nineteenth-century doctor who wrote *The Ethnology of the Sixth Sense* includes in his book this account involving a sergeant in France who said to an enlisted man:

> I bet you a pint that you and I are an unequal pair; you know
> I am talking about our things in our c ....' 'I take your bet,'
> replied the recruit. 'Then you have lost,' said the sergeant. 'I
> have only one left, the other was taken off by a bullet which a
> damned Austrian fired at me at the battle of Austerlitz. Mine
> and your two make three.' 'No, Sergeant, it is you who have
> lost,' replied the recruit, 'for I have three, and with yours that
> makes four, an equal number. Pay for the pint.'

The author adds: "And the veteran paid the pint, having lost the bet for the first time after he had won it so often."

In the present time Gore Vidal, the late noted novelist of *Myra Breckinridge* and other flights of fancy, unabashedly disclosed in his memoir, *Palimpsest* (published in 1995), that his own father had three testicles. So, reportedly, does actor Tom Arnold. Though he found fame as Roseanne's twitchy husband, no one can accuse Arnold of lacking balls. It's said he is happy to discuss his three testicles. So is rock 'n' roller Jeff Hickey, who confides that the third one "is physiologically negligible, a non-functioning half lump of vein and tissue, good for winning bar bets."

Democratic "swamp-rat" strategist James Carville told reporters in 2008 that if Hillary gave Obama "one of her *cojones,* they'd both have two." As the version suggests, it's not that Hillary Clinton has the normal two testicles, but actually *three* to Obama's one. "Nothing," remarked one writer, "motivates a politician towards self-improvement more than watching some cozy TV pundit dishing out vague, hackneyed lines about the need for more ... testicles."

In Luisa Valenzuela's *The Lizard's Tail,* an imaginary biography of Lopez Rega, Isabel Peron's Minister of Social Well-Being, the protagonist referred to as the Sorcerer is born with three testicles. Valenzuela is an award-winning noted Argentine writer of magical realism.

In another novel, *Circles,* by controversial gay author-activist Perry Brass, about the inhabitants of Ki, a "distant, tribal planet," the Same-Sex men of Ki are endowed with a third testicle called "the Egg of the Eye." It produced its own sperm, or "seed." As the author explains in his introduction: "Exchanging seed from the third Egg was at the heart of Same-Sex bonding. Seed produced intense, mystical vision. It could travel through space on its own and replicate itself."

*Les Onze Mille Verges* by the celebrated early twentieth-century poet, novelist, and advocate of modern painting Guillaume Apolinaire [Guillelmus Apollinaris de Kostrowitzky] includes this classic case of amorously assumed (and briefly mistaken) identity: Mony, "finding himself in a room even darker than the first," advances rapidly towards the sound of a female voice and comes across a bed. She murmurs: "Let's fuck. I can't wait. Naughty man, you haven't been to see me in a month." Mony climbs onto the bed and thrusts his gun ferociously into the hairy breach of the unknown woman.

At the same time, she put her hand at the root of the organ that was pleasuring her and began to stroke the two little nuts which serve as appendages and are known as testicles. The hand of the unknown woman delicately massaged Mony's balls. All of a sudden she let out a cry and, with a jerk of her arse, dislodged the ravisher. 'Monsieur!' she cried, 'you have deceived me. My lover has three!'

In the short-short biographical narrative *The Wayward Years*, the writer introduces us to his friend Mark, "who had three testicles."

As such we would usually live vicariously through his sexual exploits. It never fails at parties; mention to a girl that you have more testicles than every other guy in the room, and she's yours forever. And he would always do it so nonchalantly. He'd let the girls coo and caw over the local stud, then walk over and drop that line like it was an Ace of Spades. 'I have three balls.'

In what is surely a rare reference in a play to triorchidism, the brilliant comic playwright of ancient Athens, Aristophanes, provides an allusion concerning testicular proof of sexual potency in his best comedy, *The Clouds*. At the end of the play the Chorus sings: "Here comes your famous father, the ruler of the sea, delighted to see his three lecherous kinglets." The editor of *The Complete Greek Drama* notes that this is a pun on the Greek words *triarchoi* ["three kings"] and *triorchoi* ["having three testicles"] -- that is, endowed with 50 percent more sexuality than normal.

Triorchidism has been introduced in films as well. Close to the end of *In or Out*, a movie about a high school teacher outed on TV, one of several women making confessions concedes: "My husband has three testicles."

In *Austin Powers in Goldmember*, a continued spoof of the James

Bond films, Dr. Evil, after being accidentally struck in the crotch, says he can't feel his "balls," then puts his hand down there and ends up counting three testicles. And the hero of the enormously popular movie *My Big Fat Greek Wedding* exclaims, "I have three testicles!"

An earlier film, the 1985 kinky *E3: The Extra Testicle*, said to be one of the all-time classic pornos, concerns a green alien with three testicles "who tries to hook up with some Earth babes."

For a closing polyorchid jotting: It was reported that internationally acclaimed German artist Jonathan Meese back in 2005 fabricated a seven-foot tall 1000-pound bronze statue personifying a Russian oligarch equipped with outrageously large penises and *six* testicles.

# CHAPTER IV

# The Pleasures of Size

While there's an insatiable curiosity and anxiety regarding penile size (some would call it an obsessively searching for "the perfect penis"), the unremitting concern about sexual adequacy explains a similar absorption with testicular dimensions. A big penis fascinates; one can say the same thing about a hefty scrotum.

This is relevant not only in matters sexual. In a tactic by the Gray Davis campaign to gain advantage in the California recall election of 2003, the governor proposed the job of the state's leader be determined not by votes, but by testicle size. "I think that the job of governor should go to the guy with balls big enough to do it," said Davis. The tactic questioned Arnold Schwarzenegger's masculinity, considering "The Governator's" past steroid use during his weight-lifting days.

Four years later, in July 2007, Jon Stewart, host of the Daily Show, reminded viewers: "In D.C., they say Pat Leahy's balls grew three sizes that day." He was referring to the Vermont senator's issuing a subpoena to President George W. Bush's controversial Deputy Chief of Staff Karl Rove.

That same year Scott Raab, in his panegyrical article on Congressman Dennis Kucinich for *Esquire,* wrote that what this "warthwacked nation needs is ... a sixty-one year old vegan peacemonger

... hauling balls big enough to ... choke Dick Cheney."

The subject of testicle size is of such enormity, in fact, that as of mid-2006, Google listed 598,000 related items beginning with "Is there any way to increase the size of testicles?" Six years later, the number of entries had grown to over 2,400,000.

Yahoo! provided almost six times as many search results, yet admittedly, only a fraction of the interest in penile dimensions, about which it provided over 63 million entries by the end of 2011.

The Bulge Research Institute was created in 1992 "to research what creates a bulge in garments worn by men." Current research is focused on the size of a man's scrotum. A discussion group was formed "totally FREE for all to share stories, sightings, and/or questions about having abnormal low-hanging ballsacks or oversized nuts."

The prominent 16th century physician and pioneer in medical research Giovanni Marinello, in his advice to prospective parents, wrote: "The man who will have healthy boys is strong of body himself with ... large testicles [among other attributes]."

To achieve that, an ad in one periodical promotes an electric vacuum with a balls attachment that "will double their size." Sales conceivably have been brisk despite widely circulated warnings that any such appliance is totally without worth.

## Women's Interest in Size

The irrepressible and scandalous radio and TV "shock jock" Howard Stern in May of '97 received a call from a listener who proudly claimed to have a testicle "the size of a potato." Kevin, "The Giant Testicle Guy," was invited to the studio to "show off his hugeness." According to the Stern Show News Archives: "Howard told the guy to show him the thing, so he did. Everyone, well all of the men in the studio, went nuts when they saw the thing. Howard couldn't believe what he saw. Robin [Howard's long-time colleague] couldn't believe her eyes either." Amy, one of Stern's interns, "came in to see it but she wasn't quite as excited to see the thing."

But to show that the New Millennium Ms. is not all that indifferent to testicle size, freelancer Janice Dunn, writing for *GQ* magazine, discloses: "My friend Kira calls me after picking up a cute long hair. 'Fun night,' she says, 'But I can't get past his balls. They're tiny, like robins' eggs. I can fit them both neatly in the palm of my hand.' By the time she was done taking him down, his nads were the size of Rice Krispies. Before the milk."

A different problem was mentioned in an online Is It Normal? story: "My boyfriend has got a really big bag, you know, his balls. His dick size is about the same as other bfs have been, but his balls are huge; each one is the size of an egg. All my gfs notice his bulge and tell me how lucky I am, but they don't know it's all balls and not dick." The writer concludes, "Is it normal for a 19-year-old guy to have testicles so big?" To which one reader responds: "U haven't seen mine yet. They're like Easter eggs. My nickname is applebollox."

Another female confessed online: "I'm a 42-year-old woman who loves men with big balls! Back in my college youth, me and my friends always competed to find a male with the biggest balls. We didn't care how big his cock was. It was the size of his testicles that counted." Further along she talks about seeing "'Big John,' as he liked to be called, at a flea market — believe it or not. He was unloading a truck at a stand. I watched as he was bending over lifting an old iron stove from a pick-up. It must have weighed 300 pounds easily. His pants tightened, and I could see a huge outline of his testicles midway down his right thigh. They were as big as apples. I've seen big balls before, but this guy was the one I've been waiting for all my life. Watching as he lifted the stove up with a grunt I would see his balls pull up but not far. I almost swooned at the sight of those big testicles hanging free and loose."

She Loves Big Balls, a members-only subscription website, offers thousands of videos. One 146-image, 41-minute set features Gia, who "has one thing on her mind. Balls, sucking on your balls like they are the last pair on earth." A 129-picture, 42-minute-long video shows Crystal in action: "Tea bagging poolside anyone? The water in the pool is not quite hot enough for tea, but by the time she gets done with this guy it may just need some ice."

One 43-year-old wife writing to sex consultant Isadora Alman asks: " ... why should I be so turned on by the sight of a big set of balls? I've never heard or read about this anywhere. All I've heard is that penis size doesn't matter in sex — but does ball size heighten the sex if the man has big, low-hanging balls?"

Isadora responds:

> You are not the only one to find big balls or low-hanging ones arousing. There are leather ball pouches in sexual toy stores which enhance that look and feel. Some men even pump sterile solutions into their scrotum to enlarge them. (Do not try this at home, please.) 'Penis size doesn't matter in sex' is nonsense to those to whom it does matter. If someone finds the sight or feel of huge balls wildly exciting, sexual arousal might then be heightened with someone who has them.

Alman might have noted that one criterion the tribal Sulod girls in the Philippines have for choosing a mate is a boy's large testicles. They believe the larger the testicles, the more good luck the boy will bring to the relationship. They obviously are unaware of some startling information reported in a *Times* of London article headed "Plastic cal-lipers get the measure of the promiscuous male." From the write-up one concludes that a woman might be able to get forewarning of her partner's propensity to stray by noting the size of his testicles. Dr. Robert Baker of Manchester University explained at a conference of Britain's most eminent scientists in August 1997 that men with large testicles are far more likely to be unfaithful to their partners.

Those with testicles slightly larger than a ping-pong ball had about 30 percent more sex and more sexual partners than men with testicles the size of a large grape.

Dr. Baker had asked 80 student volunteers to his study to measure the size of their left testicle, using a set of plastic calipers supplied for the purpose. They were also asked to reveal their sexual experiences and to retain evidence of sperm volume by using condoms and recovering them without spillage after sex.

"Bad boys have big balls," was the succinct summary of the experiment by Mark Ferguson, also of Manchester University, who chaired the session in which Dr. Baker reported his results. (The average testicle size was 24 cubic centimeters [1.4 cubic inches], whilst the largest was 52 [3.1 cubic inches].)

In reporting on a more recent scientific study at Syracuse University in New York that focused on the biological relationship between bats, their testicles, and their brains, the British magazine the *Economist* casually mentioned: "Greater promiscuity does, indeed, lead to bigger testes, presumably because a male needs to make more sperm to have a fighting chance of fathering offspring, if those sperm are competing with a lot of other males." The writer, Mary Ann Sorrentino, wryly adds: "The naughtier we women are, the bigger theirs gets. They 'shrink' to embarrassing miniatures only if we are prudish."

## Small Size

For some men, diminutive testes are a cause for anxiety or a peculiar fetish. Consider these phrases in certain of the classified ads in *Small Gazette,* a 46-page quarterly aimed at those born with small genitalia and those seeking to contact them: "small mis-matched balls," "small shaved balls," "small balls, thin cock," "average endowment with small balls," "seeks men with tiny balls," "big beefy stud with small jewels."

Responding to an ad one subscriber wrote: "All my life I have always been very self-conscious because my balls are so small." Another wrote: "My balls are quite small. The right one is only ½ the size of little 'lefty.'"

Replies to a website discussion board dealing with testicular size included these follow-ups: "I am 49 years old. I have always had small testicles. It doesn't matter when your wife loves you. I always noted how large other men's testicles are. I am embarrassed to change in front of other men." And: "I am 18 years old and my testicles are pretty small, about the size of olives. Since my penis is relatively large, it completely hides my ball sack, which looks sort of strange. My girlfriend doesn't care that I have small balls, because the size of my dick makes up for it."

Laments an Internet Small Nuts Group member: "My balls on an orchidometer are about size 8-10 when they should be at least a size 16 by now. Anyway, being half the size I'd like them to be, I was wondering if anyone knows of any way to increase their size."

A *Playgirl* reader querying Dr. Joy Davidson, the magazine's "Sex Talk" columnist, asks: "My new partner's cock seemed average enough, but his testicles felt quite small. Is there any correlation to a man's virility and the size of his balls? What does the size actually indicate, if anything?"

Dr. Davidson responds: "Think of the scrotum as a warehouse containing a hormone- and sperm-producing factory. Since only a minimal amount of space is required to hold the essential production equipment, the factory needn't be large.... Small-breasted women can lactate, small-footed men can walk and run, and men with smaller genitals can be giants of virility."

Additional insight is provided by Dr. Fred Nijhout, a developmental biologist at Duke University, who has concluded that the final size of an organ is determined by an interaction between it and lots of other things in the body. In researching dung beetles, he and his associate found that the bigger a beetle's horns, the smaller its eyes, and vice versa.

But, admit the researchers, their study raises many more questions than it answers. For while their view of development looks like a zero-sum game of resources where what one body part gets, the others lose, the interaction between body parts may be more complex than that. The scientists concede there are nearly limitless possibilities for how body parts might influence each other's growth.

"Does this scientific study suggest that Ross Perot's ears were grown at the cost of another structure in his head or that Cindy Crawford's inordinately long legs mean she was shorted elsewhere?" asks the writer reporting on the investigations.

The researchers declined to comment on anyone's body parts in particular. Instead they noted that while there was no evidence that any of the more intriguing proportional anomalies in humans was caused by competition among body parts, such competition and all its effects remain possible, at least theoretically.


## Surgery

These days there's a plastic surgery procedure to renovate and rejuvenate just about anything. If women are now paying big bucks to make their privates look and feel like new (for instance, DLV — the aesthetic surgical enhancement of the vulva structure, buttock augmentation costing $6,000-$10,000, labiaplasty that reconfigures the outer labia of the vagina, hymen-reattachment surgery and "G-Spot Amplification"), and if even your neutered, cryptorchid or monorchid pet can have a silicone Neuticle implant (sizes to xxlarge starting at $94 plus the surgery), why not men?

In fact, those who covet more sizable testes can contact the Reed Centre for Genital Surgery in Bay Harbor, Florida, which advertises a procedure of testicular enlargement. "Rather than a fluff appearance of the scrotum," reads one of the clinic's ads, "the pleasing contours of two well-represented gonads are noticeable."

Dr. Harold Reed does not recommend prosthetic surgery for men with normal-sized testicles.

The physician at Reed builds the front and sides "with a crescentic soft silicone mold. Each mold is made to your unique specifications." The fee, including prostheses, local anesthesia, and the facility is $4,500 for a single implant or $6,000 for bilateral implants.

Dr. Robert H. Stubbs, the Toronto, Ontario plastic surgeon on the cutting edge of genital aesthetic surgery, reports that "a lot of American patients are coming [to see him] because we still have the solid silicone implants which are the best. They feel like a testicle, they're malleable, and they have the right weight."

The Barron Centers for Male Enhancement Surgery in Beverly Hills advertise a different technique for increasing size: namely, transferring fat to the scrotal sac. Dr. Barron cautions that "as with any fat transfer there is a significant possibility of re-absorption of the transferred fat over time."

At another Beverly Hills clinic, the Male Enhancement Center, Dr. James J. Elist implants a prosthesis into the scrotum on an outpatient basis. It comes in three sizes (medium, large, and extra large) "so that you can customize your degree of enlargement."

"The attention of the scrotum and the rational size of it in comparison to the penis and genital area have been given attention recently," acknowledges Berlin, Germany urologist Dr. Aref El-Seweifi in explaining his procedure for testicle enlargement: the implanting of a prosthesis, which gives "a new look for the organ without the feeling of having extranumerary testicles."

The MEN clinic in Chicago does a "simple surgical procedure" resulting in the scrotum appearing larger and fuller. It notes that "large testicles are often equated with manliness, power, strength, and virility." "The amount of increase," according to the clinic, "depends on the amount of fat used and this can be customized to the patient's needs and wishes." The operation takes about thirty minutes and costs $4,300.

At the Copenhagen (Denmark) Clinic for Cosmetic Plastic Surgery, Søren Hammen, head surgeon, says, "We're seeing a lot of men who, for cosmetic reasons, want bigger testicles — a relatively simple operation where we inject silicone into the scrotum." According to him, men account for about ten percent of the number of cosmetic operations performed at his clinic.

In an episode of the Emmy and Golden Globe award-winning TV medical drama *Nip/Tuck*, wealthy tycoon Burt Landau (played by Larry Hagman) arrives at a South Beach plastic-surgery clinic to get an upgrade on an earlier procedure. "It feels like I've got an SUV riding around on training wheels down there," Burt laments. He wants a pair of kiwi-size male imperatives to replace his earlier testicles.

## Other Than Surgery

Beyond the newfangled cosmetic procedures, consider the bizarre practice of the African Bubal tribe. Until they marry, the children eat the menstrual matter of cows to help fight diseases such as scurvy and leukemia. But after the males reach puberty, their testicles grow to a monstrous 28-32 inches in diameter. It is said the hormone-rich menstrual secretion of the cattle causes irreversible hormone changes in humans. "It is noteworthy," comments one report, "that such giant testicles do not exert any negative influence on the reproductive function, although they do cause many other obvious problems."

But a decidedly more normal dietary matter might deserve attention if you consider that researchers have noticed the testicles of yogurt-eating mice were five percent heavier than those mice fed a standard mouse diet and a full 15 percent heavier than those of mice forced to live on high-fat, low-nutrient junk food.

Other researchers, those at the University of Brussels, have confirmed that certain visual stimuli have a direct impact on the proportions of one's reproductive system. They found that reading certain men's magazines actually increased the size of men's testicles. Researchers found the greatest increase occurred while reading *Real Man Magazine*, "the world's most popular online magazine for the man's man."

## Size Sites

There is an abundance of websites concerned with testicular size. "When was the last time you had a chance to openly compare and contrast your ... scrotum with other men's?" asks the Images of Size site. "Here you can see over 60 pics selected to show the variability of the testicles and scrotum between men. The testicle pictures show scrotums so tight they are almost invisible, and ones so loose they are about six inches or more in length." A members-only MSN group catering to men with large testes is The Guys With Big Balls.

Several Yahoo! members-only adult interest groups are obsessively concerned with testicle size: Knackerbag, having over 3000 members as of 2012, in its home-page description remarks: "You have to admit that a big pair of bull balls, hangin' heavy and low in a loose fleshly ball sac is a fine sight to behold on a man." The Low Hangers group reminds its more than 8000 members that they can trade pics of guys "with low-hangers or otherwise beautiful or big balls."

Another group, Big Balls or Low Hangers II, founded in 2003, is dedicated "to the big balls, bull nuts and low-hanging ball lovers of the world." The results of one of its polls revealed that 23 percent of the members responding consider themselves possessors of "big, huge bull nuts"; five percent indicated "my balls are like little bird eggs."

The Fine-Jewels group polled its members: "Which size balls & sac size do you find the sexiest?" Over 40 percent of those voting checked "low hangers, large testicles." Another 24 percent prefer a "well-formed, dangling sac."

The extinct group, a9bullsballs, with a membership at the end of 2005 of 1642, was for "men with huge testicles that hardly fit into women's mouths." Another group is for women: Girls That Love Big Balls.

I've Got Big Balls, founded November 2003, claims 4029 members as of June 2011. It is "a group for the owners and admirers of big balls, low hangers, etc." Admirers, indeed: In one of its surveys 43 percent voted "big" in answering the question "How do you like balls?"

The Low Hangers group is for those with an "interest in, fascination of, appreciation for, and love of guys' balls — the very best, most beautiful, delicious, and wonderful part of the male body." Such words of jubilation call to mind Salvador Dali's own exaltation: "Of all the beauties of the human body it is the testicles that impress me most. In looking at them I feel metaphysical enthusiasm."

The 3723-member [as of 2012] Hung or Low Slung group "dedicated to admirers of the well-endowed male" urges "Ballsey Men to share with the group and feel free to show off what you're hangin' by posting your self pics in the photo section."

Rantallion.com is a "big testicle or low-hanging ball support group." Its "I Got Big Balls" forum is an "area for guys that have HUGE TESTICLES, much larger than ever, the type that cause a big bulge." The site's index includes an I've Seen HUGE Nuts section: "What did you see or witness in college? Maybe you were on a team or in a dorm. Did you see some good male meatballs while serving in the army, air force, marines, navy, or coast guard? Tell us about them. In an office, on a loading dock, in a delivery truck ... what about the balls? Ever see a low hanging sack swinging in a movie, TV show, play, or in person? Give us all the details."

The term "rantallion," in case you don't know, is an archaic expression referring to a man whose scrotum is so relaxed as to be longer than his penis. Or as defined by the Urban Dictionary, "One whose shot pouch is longer than the barrel of his fouling piece."

For as little as $5.95 at one time you could join Apple Sacks and Scrotum Farm. It provided a free preview, "but you can't see the low hanging apples unless you join." "As a member you see the real raw up-close photos of male apple sacks."

Mattersofsize.com asserts that "a larger scrotum is no longer an unattainable thing." The "natural enlargement" program marketed sells for $49.15.

But be aware that size can have a down side. Writes one IsItNormal? reader: "I have enormous balls to the point of being painful. I can't take my women from behind cause my balls slap too hard on their arses. And it's f**king agony." And someone replies, "Can you not make some sort of cradle to hold them up? Use some elastic bands and cut a sock in half."

A member of Yahoo!'s Everything_Ballz group tells of his own problem: "My balls are huge and I have a low-hanging ball-bag. They cause a lot of problems. Because of their size I wear a jock to work to help hide them, because people stare at them if I don't. I look obscene in speedos and levi's, and even with a jock strap I can't hide them."

Fridgemagazine.com announces a solution to the xxx-size problem. Writes the Fridge: "I have created my own underwear called Re-Run's Pocket Underwear for men with big balls. It keeps you front and center whether you're walking, standing, or jogging."

The Fridge, assuredly, didn't have in mind the size problem of one Wesley Warren Jr., 47, residing in Las Vegas. Due to elephantiasis, a medical condition rarely seen outside of the tropics, Warren's scrotum has grown to 100 pounds. After physicians told him the corrective procedure would cost upwards to a million dollars he set up an email address in 2011 for those who would like to donate.


## Car and Truck Nutz

Huge gonads that dangle as back-of-the-vehicle decoration are another matter. Recently a Republican state legislator in Maryland who said children shouldn't be exposed to giant plastic testicles hanging from pickup truck trailer hitches introduced on the floor of the House of Delegates a bill that, in part, "Prohibits a person from displaying on a motor vehicle a specified item that depicts or resembles anatomically correct, less than completely and opaquely covered, human or animal genitals ...." Had it passed, the offense would have been punishable by fines of up to $500. Pamela Campbell, whose Bullhead City, Arizona business sells fake bull testicles, suggested that the swinging decorations can prompt healthy discussions about anatomy and reproduction.

## Literary Utterances

Testicular size gets attention in the pages of popular literary works. In Jean Genet's *The Thief's Journal* — a self-absorbed account of a degraded past — Armand insolently boasts to Stilitano:

> 'It's my balls,' he said, 'my balls! Women walk with their tits bulging, don't they? They parade them, don't they? Well, I've got a right to let my balls stick out so people can see them, and even to offer them on a platter. I've got a great pair of balls and I've even got a right to send them as a present to Pola Negri or the Prince of Wales.'

King Samandal, in one of the accounts comprising *The Arabian Nights: Tales from a Thousand and One Nights*, had even more cause for self-assurance; we learn that when he was attacked by his enemies and fearful havoc was wrought, he flew into such terrible anger "that his remarkable testicles which usually hung to his knees, were retracted to his navel."

Size is mentioned in Philip Roth's controversial best-selling novel of 1967, *Portnoy's Complaint*. In the explicit and profane self-account of Jewish family life, Alexander Portnoy says of his father:

> Oh, thank God! Thank God! At least *he* had the cock and the balls! Pregnable (putting it mildly) as his masculinity was in this world of *goyim* with golden hair and silver tongues, between his legs (God bless my father!) he was constructed like a man of consequence, two big healthy balls such as a king would be proud to put on display....

Even the heroes of Viking Age Icelandic sagas talked about genital size. In one narrative a woman bursts out laughing when she sees Grettir Asmundarson naked. She remarks: "It seems to me extraordinary how small he is below; I would not have believed it if someone had told me." The defensive Grettir points out that his large testicles compensate for his small penis.

Bulk gets attention in less imaginative prose in a diversity of books and periodicals. For the non-explorer of the salacious, this example from the short, short story "Great Balls of Fire":

... what I saw defied description. I just stared dumbfounded at his crotch.

'Pretty incredible, ain't it,' he said, rising to a standing position. His cock dropped down and lay there in the shaft of light from the window. It was beautiful. That wasn't the extraordinary thing. But his balls! I'd never seen anything like them. They were so big and full, hanging down halfway to his knees.

'You see how big they are? I've always had a problem because of them. I thought maybe you might know what to do with them.' The irony of this last remark was not lost on either of us. 'I can't find any underwear that fits. They all scrunch up around my balls and it's killing me. I keep getting jock itch. That's why I don't wear any underwear at all.'

Inadequate proportions, comparatively speaking, get a paragraph in Michael Carson's entertaining novel *Brothers in Arms* — a story of young Benson's coming of age.

The Greek ideals were remarkable like Benson in the pubic region. Positively prepubescent, he felt. They, like him, would be giggled at in the showers for not being well developed ....

Hepher, standing toweling himself after a shower, his penis hanging like a cucumber, his slack scrotum, two new potatoes in a bag, supporting its base like a pillow, had said as much to McCarthy. McCarthy, as far as Benson could judge, resembled Benson in dimensions. Unlike Benson, however, McCarthy went into the showers in the nude, something, which, in the circumstances, Benson could just not understand. It was not really modesty which stopped Benson from baring himself to the other boys, merely a sense of shame and inferiority, a feeling that he did not match up.

## Limericks

Then, too, consider these pertinent bawdy limericks:

A long-peckered lecher named Brock
Used a barrow to carry his cock.
>    He has such massive balls
>    He can't go through halls,
And must leave them at home under lock

\* \* \*

An old Injun chief from Sioux Falls
Was known for the size of his balls.
>    "Too heavy to tote 'em,"
>    He said of his scrotum.
Wherever he goes, he just crawls.

\* \* \*

There was a young man of Devizes
Whose testes were two different sizes.
>    The one was so small
>    It was no ball at all;
But the other one won several prizes.

* * *

There was a young fellow named Thwart
Whose prick, although thick, was quite short.
    But to make up this loss
    He had balls like a horse,
And he never spent less than a quart.


## Pop Culture

Testicles of immense measure are an underlying amusement of the pop culture scene. Take the weekly comic strip "Iron Balls McGinty" featured in *Chuck Magazine*. Early on we learn: "Born without testicles, the McGinty son, Francis, faced a difficult childhood. At school the other boys taunted him mercilessly." One day McGinty senior takes his son to a circus where the boy mounts a baby elephant. Catastrophe ensues. Scared by a mouse, the animal rolls over; Francis is crushed.

In a hospital emergency room: "Dr. Patty O'Furniture, trusted friend and neighbor of the McGinty's, sees an opportunity to help young Francis — not only saving his life, but by giving him a shot at manhood with a radical procedure ... elephantoplasty." In a subsequent cartoon, Dr. O'Furniture requests: "Bring in the elephant's balls." Then he says to himself: "Someday, Francis me Boy-O, you'll be the biggest man in town." After three weeks in the hospital, "Francis finds something strange in his pajama pants: 'I've heard of puberty kicking in, but this is ridiculous!'"

Later on says the doctor to Francis: "Why, there's no telling what could happen by the time yer full-grown ... Jesus, Mary, and Joseph! What have I done?"

By age sixteen, "Not only did [Francis] have more friends, but more dates, too .... He had a new nickname, too. The kids call him 'Iron Balls.'" What follows are his adventures in Ulster with the I.R.A. (the Irish Republican Avengers).

*Viz* magazine's comic character Buster Gonads was blessed with "unfeasibly large testicles" which he was obliged to carry around in a wheelbarrow. Buster's nuts, we are told, were enlarged by cosmic rays.

Enormous testicles, though admittedly not of human males but rather, according to legend, of the tanuki — a raccoon dog native to Japan — figure in the delightful, often uproariously funny animation film *Pomoko*, released in 1994.

The feature movie by Hayao Miyazaki, justly called the "Disney of Japan," is about the efforts of the raccoons to protect their natural habitat against the encroaching city. Faced with this destruction, the tanuki fight back, using, among their mischievous devices, their large testicles as parachutes for a desperate suicide attack.

With generations of artistic freedom, Japanese artists have exaggerated the tanuki's testicles to outrageous extremes: balls that you can carry over your shoulder, drum music, or perform sumo matches on.

Among the recent crop of rappers, Grand Puba Maxwell speaks fondly of "swimming in my daddy's big nuts."

The prominent music group AC/DC sings about "Big Balls" that "should be held every night." Writes Andy Rocker about the lyrics: "It's a double meaning right until the end of the song." But there's no ambiguity about the "AC/DC I've Got Big Balls" tee shirts.

Other novelty items include the Nawty Pecker Gift Mug: "The large testicles allow for the mug to sit flat and allow for better grip," says the catalogue description.

# CHAPTER V

# The Pleasures of BDSM

Some men enjoy having their scrotum bound, beaten, kicked, stomped, whomped, chomped, punched, pinched, pistol-whipped, bashed, bludgeoned, smashed, and even ground with a mortar and pestle. "Cruelly creative body modifiers are tormenting testicles with intense neo-primitive zeal," observes Hank Hyena, a frequent Salon contributor. "Floppy flesh-sacks are getting skewed, burned, stretched, slapped, injected with liquids, and even slashed off," he adds.

## BDSM Explained

BDSM is a 6-for-4 deal of an acronym: bondage, discipline, dominance, submission, sadism, and masochism. Sometimes it's referred to as S&M, B&D, leather and fetish.

Questions about the sub-culture of organized fetishism abound. How popular is it? Alfred Kinsey found that 20 percent of the men and 12 percent of the women in his survey expressed some degree of arousal in response to sadomasochistic stories. According to professional estimates five to ten percent of adult Americans regularly engage in some form of dominant and submissive eroticism.

Are people who practice S&M "damaged" in some way? A survey that reached 20,000 people revealed that S&Mers were "no more likely to be unhappy or anxious." Another recent survey found that consensual S&M "eventuates in profound self-knowledge and transcendent levels of intimacy."

## Unrestrained Ventures

A 1987 issue of *BCQ* (*Ball Club Quarterly*) reported that the "first unofficial Ball Club convention" happened in Las Vegas in July of that year, and it announced plans for a Ball Busters' Bust — "a blatant blast, a booming blockbuster with no room for boredom" — to be held the following year at a ranch on California's northern coast. A follow-up notice listed numerous activities: a Mr. Balls contest, a guess-the-size contest, ball weight-lifting, a "Lowest Hangers Contest," and a "Tug of Balls."

The quarterly *B.B. Ads* (formerly *Muscles and Workouts*), another national periodical, in one issue carried an ad for the Huge Balls Admirers' Club and an announcement for a Balls Boxing Labor Day weekend. Participants were instructed:

> To up-lift the Balls up and out front, for punching, a heavy cloth belt 1¼" wide must be worn under the Balls. [Also] under the Balls, a foam-rubber pad, 1" thick and 4"x7" is folded over the belt and held in place by rubber bands.

> Shorts or long pants may be worn, with the front cut out to fully expose the Balls.

> Preliminary rounds will be only 15 seconds, with 45 seconds between rounds. An odd number of rounds will be 7, 11, or 15.

> The Championship bout will be 15 rounds of one full minute each, with one minute rest between rounds.

Box-gloves, at least 8 oz. weight, will be worn by Balls-Boxers on right fists during the odd numbered rounds and on left fists during even numbered rounds. You get one point for each punch your balls receive and two points for each of your punches opponent blocks.

A competition more uncommon and excruciating was recounted in the webzine Gettingit.com: "When I was prepubescent my brother Oliver and I used to maim ourselves in nutty, scorching contests. We'd press our hairless scrotums against illuminated light bulbs until one of us surrendered. Our endurance ordeals caused second-degree burns, scabbing, and dangerous layers of skin-peeling."

Similarly painful were the antics in *The Nutcracker* produced by Slave and Master productions of Chicago. An ad for the pre-recorded video cassette once distributed by Bijou Video, "pioneer of classic gay porn," stated that "This ball-busting movie charts a long session in which Master Jim carefully and methodically tortures Slave Muir's nuts with an endless procession of horrifying gadgets." " ... used on the Slave's balls are a snaffle (normally used to clamp a horse's snout), a snake-bite suction cup, a vise grip, various tools that usually engrave leather."

The video's cover design, incidentally, was vastly more provocative than the non-suggestive artwork for the first album of Scrotal Torture, the band formed in 2007, or for that of the German group Cock and Ball Torture.

## S/M Playthings

Also of Germany is Mew — not a death metal musical group, but a company offering "the most extensive collection of heavy-duty bondage gear and s/m toys." Among the scrotal devices is a "ball flask" — "a fiendish alternative to ball weights," — a hollowed-out surgical stainless-steel canister affixed to a specially designed ball collar that is attached above the male orbs. "It is intended for sophis-ticated enjoyment." Also for the well-heeled: the price is $259.

"Ballz Gag," "brought to you exclusively by the MEO-Team, where we aim to take your bondage and cbt [cock and ball torture] experiences to new heights," "is a very unique collaboration of a gag and a ball stretcher that forces your partner to pleasure you." According to the catalogue description: "One high quality leather strap slips around the back of your sub's head and another around your sack just above your balls." It adds: "This particular dynamic can lead to an interesting interchange of dom and sub roles."

Double the price are the "Ball Grabbers." The "innovative little tongs are the perfect size for grabbing one ball at a time with a rela-tively low pinching force so that use is not too painful for the victim." Adds the description: "Your fantasies can know no boundaries."

Another company retails a polished metal clamp, its "6117N Ball Crusher" for $34. "Tight or loose, that's up to you — and of course dependent on how well your man is behaving. Our Ball Crusher will make him want to really obey you. If you want to see him beg just try our crusher, and screw it down a few notches."

An acrylic crusher widely available online consists of two acrylic plates connected at the top with a hinge and separated by two 1¾" screws at the bottom of the device. The back plate has a hole for in-serting the cock and balls, or just the balls. Wing nuts are used on the screws to bring the plates closer together. You can tighten the crusher all the way, making the space only 1" wide. It sells for $52.

The one-time leading gay s/m periodical, *Dungeon Master* (pub-lished between 1979 and 1994) provided in two issues ample instruc-tions on ball torture. The writer prefaces his descriptions: "As a sadist I can say without equivocation, there is nothing in the world I find more beautiful than the look of pain as my hand is crushing his [the partner's] balls."

What follows are details concerning the use of several commer-cial castration devices used on farm animals, and genital bondage involving a "Master's hand via a leash, an immovable object, or a torture device such as a weight." "A similar result may be achieved by putting a man facing a chain link fence or similar grating. Pass his cock and balls or balls alone through the fence and then securely lock on a collar, tie with rope or somehow make it impossible for the cock and balls to be withdrawn."

The writer goes on to discuss "wrapping the scrotum in such a way that the two testicles are pulled away from each other." He continues: "Heat and cold can also provide fine torture. Chemical heat and cold packs available from well-stocked drug stores can be used. For heat alone a hot candle is good. The greater the distance the wax is dripped the cooler it is on contact."

Clamping the testicles also is detailed. "I particularly like clamps with screws or other infinitely adjustable pressure plates."

Among various other clamping devices recommended are plastic clothes pins with holes in their ends. These can be applied over the entire scrotum and then laced together with string or thin rope. Once laced together, you can pluck at the various strings and produce pain in specific areas along the scrotum.

If using clothespins, stretch out a bit of scrotal skin and let a clothespin gradually take hold, making sure the delicate tubes don't get squished.

The "Ball Torture" section of the online Deviants' Dictionary devotes a paragraph to crushing, which "can be achieved with various clamps or bandage equipment like cling film (Saran Wrap) or elastic bandages (Ace bandages)." The late Tony DeBlase, celebrated s/m authority, suggested experimenting with an inflatable blood-pressure cuff. Or how about the Electro Deluxe Humbler, hand finished and beautifully lacquered, for $159.95 from the BondageFetishStore.com. This device is made to hold the balls out back between the legs. It comes with a built-in lock and key.

## Nut Attacking Sites

Busted Nuts is a website (having nothing to do with a famous dessert or a poker prodigy) "dedicated to males kicking, punching or in some other way hurting the nuts of another male. You can submit a ball-busting experience to the Story Archives, flip through the gallery of ball-busting images or submit your picture (or that of a friend) so that you can be digitally kicked in the nuts."

The "weirdly impressive, obsessively catalogued" Anaconda Video site caters to female domination fantasies that include ball-busting. And the website Scrambled Eggs is "dedicated to the art of kicking testicles." Says its home page: "the website is concerned with F/M Domination, specifically with women hitting men in the genitals in order to disable/over-power/arouse them."

The site's introduction discusses why men like to be hit in the genitals and why women like to hit them there. What follows are four pages "for the ladies," four for men including "How and where a man can get ballbusted." Furthermore, there's a Thunder From Down Under section offering video clips of "Aussie girls crippling guys with ball crushing kicks & knees."

Included also: a confidential e-mail advice service, answers to questions frequently asked about ball-busting, the Hall of Pain — a gallery of original photos submitted by visitors to the site — and a chat room: "Your chance to chat with other people about kicking testicles."

The "For the Men" section provides the following advice for those who get involved with a girlfriend/wife/etc.:

This is without doubt the safest way of getting your kicks!

The real difficulty lies in raising the subject with your partner in such a way that they show a positive interest.

One promising way (especially with intelligent or thoughtful women) is to suggest during foreplay that sex is about power games; try to get her to be more and more dominant and give her the advantage when you wrestle or playfight.

Scrambled Eggs!!! lists almost two dozen other websites devoted to kicking testicles, including three Japanese sites. Not among the line-up is the Ball Breakers Club site, whose message page during one five-month period had 50 entries including: "Looking for busting fun in UK (Scotland). Interested?," "Sexy famous guys getting it in the balls," "Looking for Action in San Jose, CA," "Ballbusting im Stuttgart," "Hot Boots and Ball Busting."

Eighty-six percent of the more than 900 girls/women participating in a MisterPoll query marked "yes" in responding to the question "have you ever kicked or kneed a boy in his balls just for your own pleasure?" Fifty-three percent indicated they do so "Every chance I get."

One guy writing to Andrea Nemerson's alt.sex.column provided this ball-busting experience:

I was recently play-fighting with my girl friend when things got a little rougher than usual. She was trying to be playful, but she kicked me in the balls so hard that I couldn't get up. After the kick she jumped on me and kept wrestling, so she didn't notice that I was hurt. Less than two minutes later she was stimulating me with her hands. This was the best orgasm of my life. I have thought about it for awhile, and I think it was the kick in the balls that made it so good.

In her reply, Andrea advised: "If you end up really getting into this, it may be safer for you in the long run to watch some ... pros abuse the testicles of willing subjects than to become such a subject yourself."

Velvet Kick, a members-only site "for connoisseurs of the busting fetish," includes graphic descriptions of its for-sale videos: *Viva Vivian*, we're enticingly told, shows "The intoxicatingly beautiful Mistress Vivian administering her unique form of dominance and ballbusting. At times sensual, at times brutal her powerful and beautiful legs and excellent heels deliver hard thumps to a man's groin, leaving him breathless. At times she has mercy on him gently caressing balls after a brutal assault."

## Videos

BrutalCBT.com assures customers that its more than 400 hours of downloadable movies provide "a new meaning to the phrase 'she has you by the balls.' Really mean and cruel Femdoms that love inflicting pain and torturing male genitals."

If you would like to appear on camera in your very own ball-busting scene, She Fights, out of St. Petersburg, Florida, can easily make all arrangements. A basic one-of-a-kind custom clip costs $600 and includes one lovely girl and one location. Each additional girl is $300.

Voyeurs strongly recommend the wacky and enormously popular Japanese sex fetish *tamakeri* (ball-kicking) videos, especially those featuring Erika Nagai, Japan's "Queen of Adult Video" ("Extremely hot! Wish I could fuck her forever!!!"). "Loads of punters are getting their kicks out of flicks where chicks do kicks — right between the legs of naked men." There are dozens of titles. One Japanese university student remarked: "I recently asked my girlfriend if she'd kick me, but she looked at me as though I was some sort of weirdo. All I can do is watch the videos. The more painful it looks the more excited I get."

Another guy writes to the Is It Normal? site: "Ever since I can remember, getting kicked in the balls or seeing someone get sacked has been a HUGE turn-on. I often watch videos of guys getting racked by some hotties and become compelled to masturbate. And yes, I would indeed welcome any girl to swing her foot up into my nads."

While viewing a kicked-in-the-balls video — or as a metaphorical substitute — you could sip a Kick in the Balls cocktail: two tablespoons of each of the following: white rum, Midori, orange juice, and cream, and one tablespoon of coconut cream blended with ice cubes. Garnish with melon balls. To heighten the pleasure, listen to one or more tracks of Tamakeri, the brutal death metal band from Finland formed in 2007.

Unless you yourself are ever involved in a ball-busting scene, you may not even care to imagine how commonplace the activity is. Bing, the Web search engine, listed almost three million available ball-busting video sites as of early 2012. After, or in place of, your favorite sitcom, you can watch "Bitchy dominatrix women brutally kicking swollen balls," or "countless hours of exclusive videos that feature ballbusting pornstars," or "clips often showcasing unusual scenarios you would have difficulty finding anywhere else."

By the way, a few years ago on an episode of the critically acclaimed hit series *Sports Science,* a team of scientists took a close look at the impact of low blows to the testicles. A human subject volunteered to get hit in the groin with a tennis ball shot out of a canon at 50 mph as he was wired from head to toe so that a scientific answer could be obtained regarding why a low blow is so crippling.

## Tying the Balls

In his comprehensive manual *SM 101,* Jay Wiseman provides instructions involving the testes. "Many dominants, especially dominant women," he says, "find the sight of unbound genitals offensive. On the other hand, they delight in the sight of ... tightly wrapped balls." Wiseman then gives these easy-to-follow step-by-step details:

If you simply want decoration, wind and knot off a few coils between his cock and his balls, thus slightly constricting his upper scrotum. If you want him to feel more sensation, wind additional coils until the rope lightly  squeezes his testicles within his scrotum. Another way to add sensation is to wrap a few coils around the top of his scrotum, then join the free ends and run them back to front, thus separating his testicles. One way to join the free ends is to twist them together at the back of his scrotum, and continue winding as you bring them to the front. At the front, separate the ends and wind them in opposite directions around the top of the scrotum,  then knot them together (usually at the top-front of the  scrotum, just under his penis).

The Ballstie online group once queried its members: "Do you like your balls tied?" Respondents were given these choices: (1) so they still flap about; (2) tightly so they stick out; (3) so tight that it hurts; (4) so the testicles are separated; (5) so your cock is pulled back beneath your legs; (6) so your balls are twisted to the left or right; (7) so your balls turn purple; (8} all the above at different times.

One guest of the Low Hanging Support Group ("now open to the public") offers these details: "One of the sex games I used to play with an ex-boyfriend was to stand facing each other and tie our balls together with string. We both had big ball sacs, and would tie up our bollocks as tight as we could. We then stood facing each other and began wanking our poles, at the same time pulling against each other's ball sacs. We normally continued until one of us shot our load. Try it; it is incredibly horny."

## Other S/M Procedures

In his book's section "Clamping the Genitals" Jay Wiseman instructs: "You can place the clamps in a row along the line of skin running up the middle of his scrotum, or you can place one clamp directly over each testicle. (Pinch the scrotal skin, and the testicle itself). For an initial session, you probably should use only two clothespins."

Care for something more intense? View the twenty-minute video *Aching Balls*. As described in a listing of Ball Club films in *Ball Club Quarterly*: "A female dominatrix nails the sac of a 40-ish man to a tree stump and pierces both balls right through with 2 hat pin type needles."

In the same periodical a reader provides details on testicular play piercing as he himself experienced it:

My top (my wife) ordered me to watch the whole process. Next I was put into a very snug ball stretcher to pull the sac tight about my balls. The top swabbed down my balls with alcohol. Then she took a needle, popped it out of its case, and placed the point against the skin over one of my balls. Before continuing, the top gave me a little time to allow the enormity of what had been done to me to sink in. I sat there looking at the hub of the needle resting against the skin of my scrotum. I know the needle was embedded deep inside my testicle, yet I had felt no pain at all. Even penetrating the skin of the sac was painless.

Eventually she repeated the procedure on my other ball.

This time there was a tiny sting as the needle entered the skin but no other sensation. I stared at my balls, each of which was impaled by a very sharp needle.

My top asked if I was man enough to take a second needle. I told her, `Yes.` Again she placed a needle against my sac and punctured a ball with it. Then she did the other side. This was very exciting for me, and my erection got even bigger. The last needle was accompanied by a very light tug as the membrane of my left testicle was pierced.

My top told me that when I asked for the second needle in each ball I committed to the third step of the scene. She gave me a needle and ordered me to stick it into one of my balls. I was very excited and had trouble keeping from trembling. I took a deep breath to steady myself and then stabbed the needle deep into my ball. I begged my top for the second needle and quickly plunged it into my other ball. Again the piercing was done with an eerie lack of pain. We both looked at the sight of the hubs of the six needles protruding from the very heart of my maleness. It was a powerful image, and we were both very excited and aroused by it.

Finally, the top removed the needles from the skin; (because I use a lot of aspirin, I tend to bleed freely). My wife wiped this up with an alcohol swab, and it soon was stopped. She gave me a final swabbing with Betadine. Then we made love.

For additional inspiration turn to other stories — true and fictional — in periodicals and online sites catering to the leather-s/m oriented male. Here are excerpts from a serial "fantasy" in one publication:

The scrotum skin was stretched amazingly tight, so tight it was almost transparent. It glistened with sweat and antiseptic. The skin was drawn over my nuts so they looked like two round-topped sand dunes. There were ten hypodermic needles in the scrotum. In my balls, pointing in all directions, were six sewing needles in each testicle.

And in the successive installment:

He placed a camera tripod between my legs that had a piece of plywood where the camera should be. On that he put a lighted candle in a frame, then the sauce pan on the frame, and slowly cranked the pan up until my hairless nuts went in the hot liquid.

'Don't move. Just enjoy the warming effect as your nut sack fluid cooks your testicles.'

It wasn't unpleasant at all, at first, but then my nuts started to get very hot, too hot. My skin didn't hurt, but inside it seemed like there was pressure building up, like the oil was boiling my sack fluid, and that it was squeezing my nuts unmercifully. The pain began to move from my balls just like the heat was spreading throughout my crotch up into my belly, down my legs. I was moaning low in my throat when he removed the pan by lowering it.

'I don't want to cook them too fast. I want these beauties tender and juicy.'

## The Pro Scene

Kat Sunlove, who wrote an advice column for *Spectator*, a weekly sex newsmagazine, in giving an account of what she, as a commercial dominatrix (i.e., a dominant female gone pro, "a bossy female queen bee of the S&M subculture") did with one paying client mentioned: "With great delight, I tortured his ... puny balls." Another writer, Deidre Evans — also a "performer" specializing in "voluptuous chastisement" — describes one particular session: "For the next hour I would alternatively tease him with sexy advances, and kick him, hard, in his vulnerable testicles." In the same source Evans details the procedure in entertaining some of her clients:

I would strap a man down on my antique steel gyno table....
Attaching clothespins to his nipples and scrotum was a

challenge to create a spontaneous work of art in the pattern of flesh and wood. Sometimes I used pins on the hardier. When I had him decorated to my satisfaction, I would let hot wax drip on his chest and groin.

Later on she continues: "I stepped solidly on his testicles. I was rewarded with a smothered shriek."

No more shocking (or any less electrifying) is this fictional account in *The Dungeon of the Dominatrix* by Susannah Breslin, best known for her reporting for the Playboy TV program *Sexcetera* and for her *Reverse Cowgirl* blog:

'Lie down on the table,' Ilsa directed him, fastening four leather cuffs with metal loops to his wrists and ankles.

She hooked the four cuffs to a pulley above. Then, she tied his testicles with a leather thong, ran down a separate and smaller pulley, hooked it to the submissive's balls, and let go. Using a crank mounted to the wall, she raised the man into the air. He now hung suspended by his hands, feet, and balls. 'Do you like that, slave?' Ilsa asked. 'Yes, Mistress,' he replied. I'd never seen a man manipulated exactly like this before; he looked pleased. Who was I to complain? He wasn't.

BDSM once viewed as the exclusive fiefdom of creepy perverts, has become quasi-respectable, stylish, and safe. Carl Frankel, in his recent website commentary "Kinky Sex: When Did BDSM Become So Wildly Popular?" points out what's becoming increasingly obvious: "The public perception of kink is shifting to match the reality. More and more people are coming to see your typical BDSM practitioner as the man or women next door who enjoys consensual role-playing with a dollop of pain on the side (or elsewhere)."

According to Ernest Greene of *Taboo*, the monthly kink lifestyle

primer, "Most of the people who are into kink use it as a way to en-
hance conventional sexual practices." He adds, "On any given day
one million people are looking at or engaging in kink."

Greene might be underestimating. Fetlife.com, "a BDSM & fetish
community for kinksters," alone claims almost 900,000 members. Its
website lists over 40 kindred groups including one called Kick me in
the Balls. Typical of its daily messages: "Would love to give my balls
up for hard kicking, punching, smashing, and skewering. Into creative
hard ballbusting, like having my balls used for a game of darts." And:
"I'm totally obsessed with being kicked in the balls. I really love the
painful ecstasy when a women kicks me repeatedly in the balls."

# CHAPTER VI

# A Diversion: Words

Balls, as in the flippant, "Oh, balls!" As in, "They say a man with two balls will always bounce back." As in, "She hiked one ... foot into his balls." Since the 1880s, this has been a popular term for testicles, a slang expression spreading across class boundaries, used by males and females alike, in ordinary speech and in literary works, in the household as in the brothel.

It is found in song, too, as when a bunch of cross-dressers in Manhattan's Vault during Christmastime launched into a rousing chorus of "Jingle Balls" in honor of a wacky exhibitionist who had Christmas bells wrapped around his scrotum.

Shakespeare used a large variety of expressions to refer to the penis as well as to the scrotum and testicles. Punning on both its shape and its function, the scrotum is referred to as a "bag" or a "purse." The testicles are compared to ball-like items such as "billiards."

Kindred expressions abound in the linguistic world. In Spanish *huevos* and in Hebrew *betzim:* in non-biological contexts, the word for eggs. In Mexico the word's *cojones*, frequently spoken, it used to be said, by John Wayne and Reagan Administration aides, the English variation of which presumably is "gajoobies." Cuban Air Force pilots who shot down two planes by anti-Castro Cuban-Americans in February of '96 were heard on tape bragging about "taking out the *cojones*" of their victims. Commented Madeleine K. Albright, who was about to be confirmed US Secretary of State: "Frankly, this is not *cojones*; this is cowardice."

A Volkswagen ad for its GTI 2006 with a gleaming photo of the sports car and bold-lettered words "Turbo-Cojones" received complaints that the word was offensive to Hispanics, and the company had the billboards removed in New York, L.A., and Miami.

Earlier, Bob Potter, a Connecticut man in West Hartford, had been strongly urged by a city official to change the proposed name for his new Mexican restaurant: C.O.Jones. Said the official, "It was a clever wordplay, but it was just not appropriate for the standards this community espouses." Josey Vogels, Canada's favorite expert on sex, finds "los ping-pongs" — another term for balls — "amusing, but a little too cute."

Avocado is a derivation of the Spanish *aguácate*, which comes from the Nahuatl word *ahauacatl*, meaning testicle.

The Japanese say *kintama*, literally "golden globes."

The Bosnians (those persons of a former kingdom in the Balkan Peninsula) were more poetic. "O my maiden of Silaj," so went a song, "you may well weave with me: I have a spool with two coils." And she answers: "Beneath the navel sprang up the sugar melon, it is neither ripe nor green, but it first aspires to a reddish hue."

Native Hawaiians metaphorically refer to coconuts. *A! Loa 'a aku la ia 'oe na niu o Kaunalewa*, translated says, "Ah! Now you have the coconuts of Kaunalewa [once a famous coconut grove on Kaua'i]." The meaning, writes Mary Kawena Pukui, who has collected Hawaiian proverbs and poetical sayings, is: "Your worldly possessions are gone. It is an impolite saying with a play on Kau-na-iewa (hang-suspended), as if to say, 'Now all you have is a hanging scrotum.'"

Discerning a diversity of sexually suggestive symbols in nature, the Kaguru people of East Africa say *kunyika huya kusina nhungu setu singi simapinga* that is, "In the bush there are our calabashes [a tree with gourd-like fruit], some full, some partly full." What they mean, writes T.O. Beidelman, who has studied Kaguru modes of thought, is that depending upon the frequency of intercourse, a man's testicles are full or not full of semen.

Mutsuo Takahashi, one of Japan's most prominent and prolific poets, likens testicles to the "two wheels" of a cannon. Elsewhere in the same collection, he calls them a "book of wisdom."

Another contemporary poet, Cathy Song, rhapsodizing about vasectomy, comments about "a damaged eggplant after the delicate operation." In his own poem on vasectomy, Patrick O'Leary sees a variety of other similarities: "Never your most attractive feature, they now resemble plucked chickens, rotting cacti, or newborn butch marines." Poet Les Tate in his "Gifts of the Night" lyrically mentions:

And the craters of the scrotum
A crumpled dynasty
Of sun-dried grapes.

Anne MacNaughton, co-founder of the Taos, New Mexico Poetry Circus, which staged the World Heavyweight Championship Poetry Bout every summer, prefers the banal. "Acually: it's balls I look for, always." begins her descriptive ode originally titled "Teste Moanial." (For the poem in its entirety, see Chapter I.)

For still more poetic metaphors consider James Kirkup's "Little Treatise of Anatomy" — each poem corresponding with a part of a hermaphroditic body — where he makes reference to a dangling "purse of shifting values like the scales of blind justice, racked by vulva-envy, anus-angst."

Less poetic is the acronym TESTICLES (They Engineer Sperm That Is Coitally Leaked, Enveloped in Semen).

The distinctive characteristics of Afro-American vernacular speech are revealed in the vocabulary of often quaint terms for male and female body parts. In addition to the common expressions "balls" and "nuts" one researcher came across "frick and frack" in studying the special vocabulary and idiomatic usage of black teenagers living in South Central Los Angeles.

Popular expressions for the actual testicles, rather than for their container ("Tupperware for testicles. It protects something more precious than flour or last night's tuna casserole, and does so for far longer") are more common in the English-speaking world. Norwegians, on the other hand, use *pung*, meaning bag. Germans refer to the testis as a sack. In Persian, the euphemistic term is *kees-el-bedn*, meaning a bag of one's belly. *Bourse*, a French word for scrotum, refers not only to a purse or bag but also a place where merchants and bankers assemble. In the ancient Latin world *fiscus*, meaning "basket," was employed. *Bursa*, surviving all over the Romania, did not appear in a sense meaning "scrotum" until the Middle Ages.

Brazilians say *saco*: when they do so with the augmentative suffix –udo, *sacudo* "can acquire connotations of both virility and courage," writes Richard G. Parker in his scholarly and fascinating account of sexual culture in contemporary Brazil. Much like the notion of "having balls" in English, the idea of a "big sack" implies "guts" or manliness in Brazilian Portuguese, writes Dr.Parker, a professor of anthropology at Columbia University.

The term *balls* derives from *bullocks* (essentially the same word as bollocks), for centuries standard English for testicles. In 1684 the British officer commanding the Straits Fleet always referred to his chaplain as Ballacks.

In a medieval British source (1366) "bullock" referred to the leaden weight of a drawbridge. Two hundred years later, *ballocks-stones* was used apparently as a term of endearment. From the fifteenth century is this example of the word's use found in the *Oxford English Dictionary*: "I have brysten both my balok stones, so fast hyed I hedyer" ("I have burst both my bullock-stones, so fast hied I hither").

Ballocky Bill the Sailor was the name of a generously testicled fictional character celebrated in verse in the nineteenth century. Ballocky Bill's doings, mentions James McDonald in his *Dictionary*

*of Obscenity, Taboo & Euphemism*, are still recounted by rugby players, but his name is often unaccountably changed to Barnacle Bill the
Sailor.

The base word is used in such figurative expressions as "to bollix
up" -- that is, to foul up. Hugh Rawson points out in his "treasury of
curses, insults, put downs, and other formerly unprintable terms" that
the anatomical sense of bullocks/bollix is not entirely obsolete; in
Johnson County, Iowa around 1900 this ditty was heard:

Yankee Doodle had a cat,
And he was full of frolics
And all the mice and rats
That came around
They grabbed him by the bollix

An Anglo-Saxon vocabulary of the tenth or the eleventh century
includes the entry *Testiculi beallucas*, as printed in Thomas Wright's *A
Volume of Vocabularies.*

It was America's "barbarous customs" in the eighteenth century,
says Allen Walker Read in his *Lexical Evidences From Folk Epigraphy
in Western North America*, that gave rise to the verb *to bullock*; he
quotes George Grieve, an Englishman who was traveling in America
in 1780-82: "In the combats [in Virginia], unless specially preclud-
ed, they are admitted (to use their own term) 'to bite, b-li-ck, and
groudge', which operations, when the first on-set with fists is over,
consists in fastening on the nose or ears of their adversaries with their
teeth, seizing him by the genitals, and dexterously scooping out an
eye."

Then there's the phrase, "stick out like a bulldog's bollacks," when
referring to a person's protuberant eyes. Related to it: "sticks out like
a dog's balls" included in the recent *Thesaurus of Traditional English
Metaphors.*

*Balls*, standard English until the fifth decade of the nineteenth century, in February 1929 was held in the United Kingdom to be obscene. By 1931 it was permissible in print, but not in the movies … nor, one can assume, in the chambers of the US Senate. Upon learning that one Anita Hill planned to include such words as "penis" and "breast" in her testimony for the Clarence Thomas confirmation hearings in 1994, two of Washington's most savvy Democratic lawyers protested vehemently that such words would be "needlessly offensive in the decorous atmosphere of the Senate."

In 1963 Geoffrey Shurlock, punctilious administrator of the Motion Picture Association of America's Production Code Administration, wrote to Jack L. Warner, the legendary Hollywood mogul, regarding a copy of Edward Albee's play *Who's Afraid of Virginia Woolf*, which was to star Elizabeth Taylor and Richard Burton: "We are setting forth the details of this play which we consider unacceptable under the code." Among the details: "Page 47: Right Ball."

In these days of sexual candor in films, any testicular mention (and they are hardly scarce in motion pictures for general circulation) gets no more than casual notice by even the most scrutinizing and prudish local censorship board. In 1991, as tabulated by Entertainment Research Group, Inc., there were sixty-one references to balls, and, in addition, seven to nuts, three to testicles, and one each to bullocks and to apricots. During the first half of '92 the numbers were relatively similar: twenty-three to balls, five each to nuts and to testicles.

Was anyone really offended when one of the characters in the comedy film *1941*, starring Dan Aykroyd and John Belushi, says: "But get her an airplane and she'll bat your balls right out of the park"?

Even extended off-hand testicular remarks, if anything, only amuse. Take those in the script of the 1981 motion picture *Neighbors*, also with Belushi and Aykroyd:

Earl Keese to wife Enid: *I think they've a dog.*
Enid Keese: *… The dog spirit is swift and faithful.*
Earl: *I don't care. I don't want him in my garden. I don't want him*

*digging up my balls.*
Enid: (sardonic tone) *Who'd want your balls?*

Later in the film as the Keeses are entertaining their new neighbors, Vic and Ramona, this exchange:

Ramona: *Do they have any country fairs around here? You know, where they do things like see which beau has the biggest balls?*
Earl: *This isn't really country. It's more of a suburban bedroom community. The local people are in the service trades; they're not farmers.*
Ramona: *Maybe we could measure their balls.* (slight pause) *Or we could measure yours, if you like.*

A decade later *L.A. Story* was released, Steve Martin's gag-filled satire of the Los Angeles lifestyle, in which goofball weatherman Harris K. Telemacher (Steve Martin) sets out to show British journalist Sara (Victoria Tennant) how wonderful the city can be. Along the way they visit the L.A. Museum of Musicology where, among items viewed, there is a hermetically sealed jar preserving — if we can believe the label — "Beethoven's Balls."

The current universality of the colloquial expression is hinted at by that grand spontaneous craze on the Internet, the Ate-My-Balls pages. Since its initial appearance on the campus of the University of Illinois at Urbana-Champaign in 1996, the unstoppable proliferation of "AMB" was almost beyond belief. Now all but fallen out of popular Internet culture, the Yahoo! AMB listing in mid-2001 included more than 230 sites, not to mention such variations as "Martha Stewart Baked My Balls," "Mother Theresa Prayed for my Balls," and "Bill Gates Bought Our Balls." In 2010, Yahoo!'s search engine listed almost 60 million results for "ate my balls."

Just as common as the slang term is the phrase, "to have _____ by the balls," meaning to have someone at a disadvantage or in one's power. Less so is the following usage cited in *A Dictionary of American Underworld Lingo*: "It takes balls (meaning courage), to heel (assault) a screw (guard) in that stir (prison)." Poet John Ciardi in his *Browser's Dictionary and Native Guide to the Unknown American Language* offered the phrase, "Go for one's balls," meaning to gamble everything. Parenthesized Ciardi: Lose, and not much of the man is left.

The simple popular expression incorporating *balls* in the *Longman Dictionary of English Idioms* is: "cold enough to freeze the balls off a brass monkey." But there are others: *the New Dictionary of American Slang* provides this one: "tight as Kelsey's nuts (or Reilly's balls or O'Reilly's balls)" meaning very parsimonious or stingy.

The term can be used, according to British etymologist Eric Partridge, to describe a dominant woman in the home: "She's the one with the balls in that family." (Former British Prime Minister Margaret Thatcher — the "Iron Lady" — was always reputed to be "the one with the balls in her marriage.") Or take these Partridge gleanings from some British periodicals: "Deke [Arion] says she'll get there [to stardom] because she's got what the greats have all got, balls 'Liza's got balls; Streisand's got great balls, hasn't she? Well, so's this lady.'" And, "It's probably one of those civil servants again, leaking (news) to the defense correspondents, just to show they're in on the act and have got balls as big as aircraft tyres."

Partridge underscores the obvious: the slangish use of "balls" in all senses derives — "however inappropriately" — from the low Standard English equivalent of testicles. In the United States it's been used colloquially for courage or "guts" since about 1935. "Courage in a woman is assumed to be rare, remarkable and no part of her FEMININE nature. It is clearly an absurd and pejorative term when used of a woman," comments Jane Mills in *Womanwords: A Vocabulary of Culture and Patriarchal Society*.

The term "to ball," it is said, has actually nothing to do with testicles, as is generally thought. One theory is that the word in this sense comes via the French *bal*, from the Latin *ballare*, meaning to dance. But it's been also said that "balling" is a "slightly more tender term" used for "fucking," with the provision that the balls be appreciated as a part of a penetrating organ.

Oddly, in Partridge's comprehensive glossary of slang words and phrases in the British armed forces, 1939-1945, not a single expression for testicles is included, other than *bullocks*, which was used to refer to the Royal Marines. Nor did the prolific lexicographer list any slang word for penis, but did include one for anus.

"Cods," another slang expression for human testes, appears in Ken Weaver's *Texas Crude*: "That fool reached for my quarter on the pool table and I kicked him in the cods twice and had the balls racked and broke before he quit pukin'."

Euphemistic expressions provide us with one way out. They are words you use out of fear or delicacy to avoid giving offense. Those referring to testicles and scrotum are so wide-ranging as to include the four major food groups: fruits and vegetables, nuts (of course) and grains, meat and fish, and dairy products.

A rich and diverse lexicon of more than 200 terms is given below. For variety's sake you can use a different one daily for over half a year without a repeat.[1]

---

1 (A) agots, acres, Alls-bay, almonds, apples, apricots, Arabian goggles (B) baby batter maker back wheels, bag of fruit, bag of tricks, bags, The Balkans, ballbag, ball sac, bangers, basket, baubles, bean pods, Beecham's Pills, berries, billiards, bird's eggs, bobbies, bobbles, bogga, bogs, bollocks, bongos, booboos, boolies, boosters, boulders, boys, brains, bullets, bum-balls, bursa virlis, buttoms (C) cahoones, callibisters, cannon balls, Charlies, charms, cherries, chestnuts, Chicken McNuggets, chumblies, churns, clackers, clangers, clappers, cluster, cobblers, cobbs, coconuts, codlings, coffee stalls, coolers, coolies, cooligans, cooyons, crackerjacks, creamballs, cream crackers, crown jewels, crystals, cubes, cullions, culls, come/cum factories, cuts (D) damsons, danglers, Davina McCalls, diamonds, dingle berries, ding-dangs, ding-dongs, do-dads, doohickeys, dobblers, donkey omelets, doodads, dowsetts, dusters (E) eggs, eggs in the basket, essentials (F) family "J's", family jewels, family treasures, flowers and frolics, fluid friends, Fred and Ethel, fries, future (G) garbonzos, gingamabobs, glands, gonads, gongs, goolies, gooseberries, grand bag, groin (H) hairy beanbag, hairy conkers, hairy saddlebags, hangin' tanks, happysacks, higgumbobs, hind legs (I) innominables (J) jatz crackers, jelly bag, Jenny Hills, jewels, jiggumabobs, jigglies, jingleberries, jocks, John Waynes, johnny rollics, The Jonas Brothers, juice crew, jumbucks, jungleberries (K) kanakas, kelks, knackers, knockers (L) ladies'jewels, lam pah, lads, leerodies, load stones, love apples, love grapes, love nuts, low-hangers, lunch, lurn, lust cluster (M) magazines, male mules, man balls, man sack, maracas, marbles, marriage gear, marriage prospects, marshmallows, Mephistopheles' purse, monster balls, monsters, mountain oysters (N) nackers, nadgers,

Considering what we hear in films these days, it seems inconceivable that during earlier decades testicular vernacularisms were verboten. The Hays Office — Hollywood's self-imposed board of censors in existence from 1934 to 1968 — decided that "nuts" was among forbidden words.

When Joseph Breen, who at one time headed the censorship rules office, wrote to a producer that a film based on this book or that play could not hope to receive a seal of approval, "A vaultlike door slammed shut."

Writing to Louis B. Mayer of MGM in 1935 about the script for *A Night at the Opera* Breen said, "We call your attention to the following ...: Page 18; The expression 'Lichee nuts to you,' should be changed ...."

July 2, 1940 Breen had received from Universal Studios the first 75 pages of *The Bank Dick*, and he had a long list of amendments to suggest. Among them: "Scene 90: Please eliminate the expression 'nuts to you' from Egbert's speech." A short time later concerning *For Whom the Bell Tolls* Breen requested: "The expression 'And nuts!' (on page 108 of the script) must be omitted."

Among other testicular expressions is "family jewels" — "a man's most valuable possession and the pride of his family, since the testicles provide progeny." "Within my own memory," wrote Partridge, it "goes back to the 1920s; what's more it smacks of educated Edwardian raffishness."

Notwithstanding, the expression is, or at least at one time was,

---

nads, nags, nards, necessaries, nerts, Niagra Falls, nicknacks, nogs, nuds, nuggets, nutmegs, nuts, nutty buddies (O) onions, orbs, orbs of love, orchestra stalls, orchestras, orchids, orks, ornaments, oysters (P) package, painter's eyes, partners, peanuts, pebbles, peeps, penis pillow, pig's knockers, pills, plums, pods, poke, potatoes, pouch, pounders, prick pals, prunes (R) raisin bag, razoos, rocks, rollies, rollocks, royal jewels (S) sack o' nuts, saddle bags, satchel full of yarbles, scalloped potatoes, scrote, seals, seedcase, self adjustment dials, scum bag, seed factory, seeds, sex glands, slabs, slashers, sperm tanks, spuds, spunk holders, squirrel food, swingers (T) tallywags, tarriways, tassel, taters, tatties, teabag, testiculus, testes satchel, testimonials, testosities, the boys, thingmajigs, thingummies, Thor's twins, Tom & Jerry, Tommy Rollocks, tool bag, trinklets, twins, two-piece, two veggies (V) velvet orbs, vitals (W) wad hammock, wank tanks, wedding kit, wedding tackle, whennymegs, winky bag, Won Hung Low, wrinkles retainer (Y) yarbles the one and only testicular colloquialism in the Aggie vocabulary of more than two hundred slang words and phrases compiled in 1946 by Fred Eikel, Jr. The "Aggie fraternity," that is, the present and former students of the Agricultural and Mechanical College of Texas, had, according to Eikel, its own vocabulary, "and it is through this vocabulary that the Aggie spirit is nurtured." He admits that some of the references are general military or college slang, while many are unique to the Aggies.

Previously the CIA used "Family Jewels" to denote internal and potentially embarrassing secrets that the agency preferred never to be disclosed to the public.

From the Ozarks comes this report: "Sharpening his knife to castrate a hog, my neighbor said, 'I'm fixing to take the weights off 'n him'." The correspondent adds: "A boy at Pineville, Mo. was threatening one of his schoolmates: 'If you monkey with me,' he shouted, 'it'll be your old tomatoes.'"

Among the whimsical testicular analogs mentioned in James T. Henke's delightful collection *Gutter Life and Language in the Early "Street" Literature of England* is bandoleers — literally the small pouches on the belt that were worn by soldiers to carry charges for muskets, but continually likened to testicles loaded with seminal "bullets."

In "The Young Damsel's Courage and Conquest," a late seventeenth-century ballad, the lyrics are an extended double entendre that belabors the equation, copulation = war. Here the maiden is victorious for

... he did shoot, the
dispute held while he'd spent his Ammunition [i.e.
seminal "bullets"]. Now his Bandillers [sic] being
empty at last so he no longer could stand the Field.

The Latin diminutive of testis is *testiculus*, from the ancient

Hebrew practice of administering the most solemn oaths by placing the hand of the testator on the testicles. It is said the custom came from Egypt where Arab men desirous of saluting or making a promise with great solemnity put their hands to the generative parts of their body. Allen Edwards corroborates this in his historical survey of the sexual culture of the East. He writes that the Arabs pledged, "I swear upon the cullions of Lord Mohammad!" Each man would then touch his secret parts and murmur: "O Father of Virile Organs, bear witness to this solemn oath!" The Hindu practice was much the same, says Edwards: Upon gripping the testes with the right hand of purity, each man would say, "We are bound together by the Salt!"

To add further confusion to the etymological matter, British lexicographer Michael Quinion on his website pointed out that *testis* derives from an Indo-European word for the number three. "That was because the Romans regarded a witness as what we would call a trusted third party, one who stands aside from the dispute and can tell it how it really was."

John Davenport points out in his discussion of the "Symbols of Reproduction," that the low Irish in Dublin and the London street sellers of fruits and vegetables, in order to give added force to an assertion, would conclude, "S'elp my taters" or "So help me testes" — equal to saying "I swear by my member." Davenport notes that the word "taters" is a corruption of, and vulgarism for, testes.

*Spermary* rather than *testicle* is a better designation as it corresponds with ovary, but it is used for certain animal groups, chiefly insects.

The obscene word in Latin for "testicle" was *coleus* (etymology obscure), which occurs in epigram but not in satire. There were, according to J.N. Adams, in his book *The Latin Sexual Vocabulary*, circumstances in which "obscenities were not tolerated by the educated."

The Greeks use the term *orchis*, which inspired Theophrastus (d. 287 B.C.), Aristotle's successor as head of the Lyceum, to apply the word for the botanical term orchid, in his *Enquiry into Plants*. It was not by mere chance, reasons urologist Charles Montgomery Steward, M.D.,"that the loveliest and most treasured flower that grows and the male gonad should have the same name." According to him, the "Father of Orchidology" probably originated the term *orchid* for *orchis* in allusion to what he saw as a similarity between the paired, enlarged underground bulbs and the testicles of humans — "a pair of fleshy tuberoids."

On the authority of a popular seventeenth-century English publication, all the species of the plant *orchis* excite the "venereal appetite" and aid in the conception because of "their similitude of the Testicles" and because "they also have the odour of the Seed."

Centuries before Theophrastus, Confucius (551-479 B.C.) is quoted as having said that "Acquaintance with good men was like entering a room full of lan, or fragrant orchids." Three hundred years after him, the Greek surgeon Dioscorides wrote in his *De Materia Medica*, for fifteen centuries the standard authority in medicine and botany, that the orchis roots influenced sexual phenomena. An infusion of the younger and firmer of these two "bults" was believed to stimulate production of a male child.

Until such a time when evolution might determine that having two genders is no longer an advantage, when an asexual female will arise, generating twice as much of herself, swamping the scene with her genes, thus wiping males off the map, (after all, there are far more efficient ways than sexual congress of reproducing oneself — no molecular barrier prevents fish, amphibians, and insects from making the switch to asexuality), the list of figurative terms for the testes is bound to grow: entirely new and innovative cyber-slang and yet-to-be-created portmanteau words.

# CHAPTER VII

# Solo Pleasures

A member of the unequivocally named Low Hanging Balls Support Group, claiming over 15,000 registered users, exuberantly confides: "When I come back from the gym — no shower taken — I love to have my smelly running shoes tied by the laces at my sack." He adds: "I get so hard."

Another guy writes to this author about "coming while having weights hung from balls. Really intensifies it for me. Have done this for some years."

PassionVillage.com's Michael Simpson details his own rapturous experience with testicle-directed solitary sex, so-called ball jocking:

> The application of lube was my introduction to ball jocking. I started massaging my testicles directly. Interestingly, when I had a hard-on it felt like my penis continued through my ball sac, to disappear at the lowest point of my hip bone. Something I had not noticed before. As I cupped and massaged my balls in my hands it seemed natural to concentrate more on this new part of my penis that had previously been unchartered. There was definitely something there, some stirring, teasing feeling waiting to come forth. It just needed patience and a little more lube.

As I worked and built this new deep feeling, my balls were there and mixed up in the action, .... It was difficult to resist the temptation to touch my penis. Time passed, five or more minutes. The longer I worked, the more I felt that my patience would soon pay off.

The final blast seemed to spread from the base of my balls to surround my entire hip region. It gripped my body for what seemed like a long time, and as I ejaculated I lay stunned, trying to decide what had happened. My orgasm had been very heavy and very deep, missing my penis completely.

Comparing it to conventional masturbation is difficult, so I am still not sure if the experience was superior, much less 'psychic.'

You decide.

Offering "Sex Fun and Wisdom," Dr. Susan M. Block salutes "Happy Masturbation Month":

When our forefathers testified, they put their hands on their testicles. *That's right*, they swore by their family jewels! Telling the truth (for a man) was assured by the public act of squeezing, stroking or gently cupping one's sac. So do like your ancestors, do like your Old Father Abraham, grab your balls and testify! Grab 'em right now, Brother! Don't grab 'em too hard. But don't be too soft on yourself either.

With exultation Block continues: "Feel the power, the glory and the truth of solo sexual revelation. Finger yourself with joy! Stroke yourself with rapture. Surrender to self pleasure. Testify to the truth of autoerotic ecstasy."

"What's your favorite way to start a masturbation session?" asks JackinWorld — The Ultimate Male Masturbation Resource. A nineteen-year-old responds: "I like to start out by slowly rubbing between my thighs, imagining there is someone down there doing it for me. Then I usually play with my testicles, slowly enjoying the feel and pleasure it provides. Usually this way of starting a session guarantees it will be a good one."

## The Tao Method

A male masturbation technique concentrating on the testicles is a part of Taoist meditation. Taoism is defined variously as a ritualistic religion, a philosophy, a Chinese folk religion, or a series of health practices similar to yoga. Over the centuries the many branches of Taoist teachings have grown, all aimed at integrating the various activities of one's daily life with the Tao.

Its testicle meditation calls for cradling the testicles in the palm of the hand, stroking them lightly to warm them up until you begin to get aroused. As you inhale, you're to gently pull upward with the muscles around the testicles, perineum (the region between the scrotum and anus in males), and anus. You are told to imagine that you are channeling your sexual energy and sexual warmth from your testicles, through the perineum, past the anus, over the tailbone, and up the back of the spine to the base of the skull.

## Other Modi Operandi

AdvancedMasturbation.com, a non-pornographic documentary resource containing masturbation information, techniques, methods, illustrations, instructions, pictures, and videos, includes an index of no fewer than forty-seven easy-to-not-so-easy techniques: three involve the scrotum.

Number 28, scrotum masturbation deep testicle massage, is

called an "advanced" technique requiring lubrication. It allows you to masturbate the scrotum while whacking off the penis at the same time. "The trick to perfecting this technique is to use the thumb and forefinger to slide along the back of the penis and all the way down to the back and underside of the scrotum."

Number 37, glass balls masturbation, involves using a drinking glass to stimulate the testicles and perineum areas as well as the anus. Sit on the very edge of a bed and let the testicles hang over the edge. Use a simple and quick up and down jerking method while holding the glass against the area underneath the testicles just so they dangle onto the edge of the glass. As a variation, you can lean back on the bed a little and use the glass to put pressure farther back, in the area of the anus. One viewer recommends, "Make sure you are naked; this adds to the fun."

The last method involving the scrotum is called the ice cold, golden testicles technique ... another "advanced" procedure. Lie on a bed with an ice cube under the testicles. Jack off until you are about to reach orgasm, while leaning back and not letting the testicles bounce off the ice cube. The website offers an alternate method: "If the ice cube on the testicles is too intense during the masturbation, simply chill the other hand with the ice cube before or during the session. Then when you are about to ejaculate, simply put the other cold hand right up against the testicles."

"Playing Ball" is one procedure described in another tips for masturbation site: "In this one you get to scratch at your balls. Gently scratch your fingernails over the surface of your balls. Alternate between doing this and massaging gently around the area surrounding each ball individually. Try tossing them around allowing them to roll slightly in the scrotal sack."

An unconventional technique mentioned in an anonymous post on solotouch.com leads to "fantastic orgasms/ejaculatory gasping-for-breath satisfaction":

Fill the first two inches of a condom with sufficient lubrication to cover well the business end of your cock.

Roll the condom to the base of your cock so that it is fully unrolled. Now stretch it over your entire scrotum enclosing both testicles. Carefully slip each testicle out of the bag so that a "roll" of your scrotum remains held in the condom. Now rub your cock to spread the lubricant evenly over it. Start and continue to slowly slide the condom up and down. Each up stroke pulls the scrotum flap and gently shakes your balls until the urge to speed to a wonderful out-pouring becomes irresistible.

Scrotal masturbation is clearly reflected in the slang phrase "to play pocket billiards." Noted psychoanalyst Dr. Jules Glenn years ago said he believed analysts had neglected the importance of sensations arising from stimulation of the testicles and scrotum. "There is," he wrote, "both a primary pleasurable aspect to the phenomenon as well as displacement from the penis. Testicular pressure, producing pain, serves to evoke masochistic gratification."

## Needles

Inserting needles into the scrotum may not be as rare you would like to believe. "I have a fantasy of having needles right into the testicle," admits one member of the Everything_BALLZ Yahoo! adult group. Another member cautions that "you need to make sure everything is sterile — skin and needle." He writes:

I found the E string on a guitar makes an excellent needle.

When you cut it at an angle this leaves a very sharp point; entry is easy. I get the feeling as it passes through the nut itself like you get just before you cum. It is awesome to see the wire come through both nuts and out the other side. You can tug on both ends of the wire or move it back and forth, or if you have left it long enough you can run it back through to the other side. I have done this too many times to count.

Stranger than fiction? Consider a scene in the intense and unsettling horror flick *Neighborhood Watch* (2005), "THE most disturbing movie ever made": Character Adrian Trumbull, "ranking definitely among the vilest psychopaths in horror cinema history," masturbates by sticking hypodermic needles in his scrotum.

## Self Ball-Busting

By mid-2012 Bing search engine was listing a mere 3,580,000 pages, images, and information on this fetish. By contrast, Yahoo! was providing three times as many results. Included was a listing for its adult Self Buster group, founded in 2001. "Let's face it," comments the group's website, "95% of BB fans don't have anyone to bust them, so a great way to feel that sweet pain is bust your own." It requests: "Leave anything to do with self-busting such as tips/advice, stories, or pictures."

A "junior member" of FemaleDom.com Ballbusting Forums writes: "While nothing can be compared with being busted by a hot girl, there are times in life when this isn't possible. So if I don't want to just think about it but actually feel the pain I guess there's only one option: self-busting."

He asks readers for technique suggestions. One member recommends dropping a toilet seat on your balls. "Just inset balls properly; watch that it can free drop and slam it down."

For less unconventional approaches, look at self-busting videos. BallbustingTube.com provides almost two dozen of them. In one, Vittoria ("this sizzlin' hot Italian babe") instructs you on how to bust your own balls. "It's the best thing next to actually having her there in the room with you stepping on your nuts." (B-B with a partner is explored in Chapter V.)

Other ideas on self-abusing the "turkey wattle bags" are shared by the thousands of members belonging to the more than 130 online ball-busting forums.

One question in a survey offered by the expansive Kramtoad's Ball Busting website asked, "What's your favorite way to bust your own nuts?" Some replies: "I usually slam one of my Nikes into them," "I cup my balls in one hand, then I punch them lightly and then squeeze them, and then punch again," "Rope bondage and/or a vise," "A juggling ball in a sock is great, and there's something called a bodystick (a rubber ball that's attached to a flexible plastic handle) that's great as well."

"One guy recently sent two tapes of his self-recorded Solo Sex. He got signed up immediately by Palm Drive Video to star solo in the not-yet-released *Ball Puncher,*" wrote Jack Fritscher in an article for *Drummer*, the sensationalist, now-defunct gay leather magazine. Fritscher continued:

> He's a traveling salesman and spends every night alone, but not lonely, in a different hotel room, videotaping himself, surrounded by décor that ranges from Motel 6 to Hyatt Regency. His Solo Sex trip is Ball Busting. Nightly, he thumps his nuts, hung over ever-changing bathroom sinks, with rubber mallets, wooden clubs, and Everlast fast-bag boxing gloves, until he shoots from his sizeable 9-inch cock. He's an artist of Solo Sex.

## Other Maltreatments

"I really love abusing each of my old pain berries directly," wrote a 63-year-old Everything_BALLZ member. "I don't do anything suddenly like hitting them, but rather I totally enjoy a long hard squeeze or a mechanically applied crush." He added: "I've come to like several different types of squeezing devices, especially locking mechanical clamps like a vise grip and constant pressure spring or stretched rubber devices that I can apply for long periods directly onto my balls after I separate them from each other with several wraps or metal rings. A pair of lobster claw rubber bands applied on each berry gives a wondrous feeling."

## Electro-Stimulation

Erotic electro-stimulation (also known as E-stim or EES) is "a wonderful way to add some new fun to your sex life," writes D. Williams, MD, for his online *Guide to Erotic Electrostimulation*. Not to be confused with the more sadistic or painful application in BDSM, it involves low-frequency electrical stimulation to the nerve and muscle tissue of the body using a power source and electrodes. According to one sexual stimulation products manufacturer, using its devices "add a new dimension to masturbation, foreplay, or intercourse." Newcomers are urged to research the hazards, limitations, and techniques of E-stim.

"There are now legions of sensualists who've discovered electricity is the best sexual enhancer since the advent of birth control," blissfully comments Michael Lane in writing about Dant'e Amore's Paradise Electro Stimulations, Inc., reputed to be "the world's foremost authority in research, development and manufacturing of erotic electro-stimulation toys." Headquartered in Las Vegas, it is one of three major manufacturers of power sources in the US.

Among power box accessories that interest us here is the testicle tubular electrode. It is designed to conform to the soft tissue mass of the scrotum, while at the same time encapsulating each testicle separately. Instructions for using this device: (1) lubricate the scrotum using electrode gel, (2) grab above each testicle, making sure the skin is smooth and tight around each testicle, (3) place the testicles, one at a time, through the conductive loops, tightening each loop, and (4) move the "O"-ring into a locking position to ensure a snug fit.

It's said with this e-stim accessory "shocking sex can be fantastic sex."

There is also the electro-stimulation scrotum parachute: a soft rubber parachute-style scrotum stretcher. Once plugged into a power box, the numerous contact points inside the parachute run "a pleasurable current through the balls, creating intensely erotic sensations."

The scrotum electrode is said to provide "a unique sensation" to the scrotal area. Its advantages are said to be in its cloth construction, which allows for comfort even during long periods of use. According to the European manufacturer, "it is also shape-conforming to the scrotum sack which allows for increased focusing capability maximizing the Erotic Electro Stimulation effect."

Kcballwork, a one-time adult Yahoo! Group, while cautioning that "involuntary muscular contractions can cause serious damage to the spermatic cord by stretching and possibly separating it from the testis," provided these pointers: "Set the electro-stimulation unit to 'thump' mode at the slowest cycle setting. The person at the control [perhaps you yourself] can now vary the voltage from a low and soothing 'tap' to a high and unbearably painful blow that will induce the unmistakable nausea of being kicked in the jewels."

The group's site called attention to the several electronic muscle stimulators (EMS) on the market. They range in price from as little as $29.59 to over $1,300 for a Globus Genesy 1100 electronic muscle stimulator.

## Free-Balling

Another solo enjoyment deserving attention here is so-called free-balling (said of a male going without supportive underpants), thus allowing one's balls to hang free and unencumbered. An additional term could be "dangling," since only men can dangle freely.

When JustUsBoys.com polled its members, "Do you free-ball?" 14 percent answered "All the time"; another 55 percent said, "Sometimes." When it asked, "Does freeball keep you in a constant state of arousal?" 37 percent of the respondents said, "Yes."

"I've been freeballing since I was 10 years old (I'm 47 now). I love to feel my balls hanging low and swinging free," comments a member of the Everything_BALLZ Yahoo! adult group. Another member confides: "I've been free-balling from around 1986 on. It's the best feeling and no restrictions."

"I love freeballing the most," jubilantly exclaims a member of The Freeballers Forum — The Art and Science of Going Underwearless. "Your balls flopping around, and how comfortable it is, and only you know there is nothing underneath — that little special secret to yourself anything you do or anywhere you go."

A fellow freeballer writes to the forum: "I got some big low hangers, too (they hang a little over five inches); I just use some talcum powder each morning, and that keeps the boys happy and dry and bouncing in my jeans or shorts all day."

In surveying its members, Freeballers Forum asked, "Do you like others to notice that you're freeballing?" One guy responded irrefutably: "Hell yeah."

Another freeballer responding to the forum survey wrote: "Since college I've spent lots of time freeballing on weekends. Just out and about, but I've recently just started to go commando more and more. In fact, I've only worn underwear to work one day this week — and HATED it. I'm hanging free in a suit for the first time today and absolutely LOVE it. It's like, oh brave new world!"

To the question "Do you freeball for the comfort or because it's daring?" he responded: "There is a definite thrill to having a secret." When asked if his "above average" balls influenced his starting to freeball, the answer was, "Yes."

MisterPoll directed the following query to freeballers ("Str8 Dudes

Only"): "Basically, do you like a guy to see your package?" Among the more than four thousand replies: "Yeah, makes me feel proud," 15%; "Yeah, it's kind of a turn on," 14%; "Yeah, definitely a turn on," 12%; "No, that's gay," 5%.

Another MisterPoll survey asked, "What type of pants do you freeball in?" Of the 524 voters responding: jeans 79%, athletic shorts 71%, dress pants 40%, dress shorts 36%, kilts 15%.

Presumably wearing dress pants, the indomitable Johnny Weir, US national figure skating champ, speaking at the recent Human Rights Campaign Seattle's annual gala dinner, nonchalantly said, "I usually try to freeball it when I give a speech like this."

So in fashion is the idea of freeballing, the use of the word ranges from a line of men's jeans and shorts available from an Australian on-line shop to the title of over 150 songs including one by well-known parody song producer Bob Rivers: "Wearin' almost nothing, gonna swing my nuts awhile ...."

## Other Delights

Someone has blissfully announced that "now you can fondle your balls in public without fear of prosecution" after seeing a life-sized model of the scrotum and testicles made from BIOLIKE synthetic tissue. One happy customer reports: "One of the best purchases that I've ever made!" Another remark: "Whoever thought pleasure lying below the belt might as well be an out-of-the-body experience. Cool."

The only downside is that the model made for teaching testicular self-examination has two synthetic tumors embedded in each testicle "seriously undercutting the warm, reassuring feeling that comes with juggling one's balls." The price: $161.70 including handling and shipping -- and a carrying case.

In any event, using this "latest innovative technology" from Canada with lustful intent would be nothing grossly improper or offensive, in contrast to some of the notorious but nonetheless self-gratifying acts at the 1991 Tailhook gathering in Las Vegas. Often groups of aviators were seen milling about in their suites or in hallways with the testicles exposed, but acting as though nothing was happening. Some would casually introduce themselves to women and mingle with them until they noticed. A popular T-shirt sold at the convention read: "If You Got 'Em, Hang 'Em."

This final thought: Let's not overlook whatever pleasure one might experience from that complex emotional and intellectual state of mind referred to as masculine self-image. One component of this has been named "egotesticle" — the belief, according to one definition, that the whole world is centered around one's testicles.

www.ingramcontent.com/pod-product-compliance
Lightning Source LLC
Chambersburg PA
CBHW020310290526
45784CB00003B/1445